TRUST YOUR BODY!
TRUST YOUR BABY!

TRUST YOUR BODY!
TRUST YOUR BABY!

Childbirth Wisdom and Cesarean Prevention

Edited by Andrea Frank Henkart

Forewords by Nancy Wainer Cohen and Michel Odent, M.D.

Bergin & Garvey
Westport, Connecticut • London

Library of Congress Cataloging-in-Publication Data

Trust your body! Trust your baby! : childbirth wisdom and cesarean
  prevention / edited by Andrea Frank Henkart ; forewords by Nancy Wainer Cohen and
  Michel Odent, M.D.
      p.   cm.
  Includes bibliographical references and index.
  ISBN 0–89789–294–1
    1. Natural childbirth.   2. Cesarean section—Prevention.
  I. Henkart, Andrea Frank.
  RG661.T775   1995
  618.4'5—dc20   94–30915

British Library Cataloguing in Publication Data is available.

Library of Congress Catalog Card Number: 94–30915
ISBN: 0–89789–294–1

First published in 1995

Bergin & Garvey, 88 Post Road West, Westport, CT 06881
An imprint of Greenwood Publishing Group, Inc.

Printed in the United States of America

The paper used in this book complies with the
Permanent Paper Standard issued by the National
Information Standards Organization (Z39.48–1984).

10 9 8 7 6 5 4 3 2 1

To my greatest teachers, my children, Journey and Quest. You are my miracles, my mirrors, my windows of life. May your children be born in the intense, emotional, joyous, sexual, loving experience that birth is. I pray you will be open and willing to accept it in its fullness.

Katie's Poem

We did it!
I yelled
We did it!

Because we knew
It was right.
You won't cut me
Not again, ever!

My baby knew.
My husband knew.
My heart knew.
Now the whole world can know.

They didn't fool me
With their jargon.
They didn't fool us
With their threats.

It was my responsibility.
It was my baby's birth.
Now, it's my joyous memory
And a part of who I am.

By Esther Booth Zorn, founder of International Cesarean Awareness Network, Inc. Reprinted by permission, 1983.

Contents

Foreword by Nancy Wainer Cohen   xi

Foreword by Michel Odent, M.D.   xv

Acknowledgments   xvii

1. Great Expectations   1
   Andrea Frank Henkart

2. On the Cutting Edge   13
   Andrea Frank Henkart

3. Ritual in the Hospital: Giving Birth the American Way   25
   Robbie E. Davis-Floyd

4. Preparing for Labor and Delivery   39
   Andrea Frank Henkart

5. Accept the Process: A Commentary on
   Childbirth Education   59
   Gina Maria Alibrandi

6. Visualization Techniques for Relaxation   67
   Andrea Frank Henkart

7. Body Wisdom: The Forgotten Information
   in Childbirth   73
   Donna Germano

8. When Push Comes to Shove: What to Do if You
   Have a Cesarean   81
   Andrea Frank Henkart

9. Healing Cesarean Section Trauma:
   A Transformational Ritual   91
   Jeannine Parvati Baker

10. One Birth at a Time   99
    Andrea Frank Henkart

11. The Husband's Role in Pregnancy   109
    John Gray

12. Birth Stories from around the World   117
    Andrea Frank Henkart

13. A Balinese Cesarean Story   127
    Robin Lim

14. Parenting the Precious Newborn   131
    Andrea Frank Henkart

15. Circumcision: A Question of Protecting Body Rights   141
    Marilyn Fayre Milos

16. A Womb of Love   151
    Andrea Frank Henkart

Appendix A. Questions to Ask Your Care Provider   155

Appendix B. Ideas for Your Birth Plan   157

Appendix C. Affirmations for Childbirth Preparation 160

Appendix D. Things You Can Do to Avoid
             Unnecessary Cesareans   162

Appendix E. Sources of Further Information   165

Bibliography and Suggested Reading List   169

Index   175

Foreword
Nancy Wainer Cohen

We hear frequently that the birth of a new baby has a profound effect on not only that mother and baby but the rest of the family—and in turn, the community and society at large. As a result, we say we understand how important it is that the woman, her pregnancy and the birth be treated with honor, respect, gentleness, caring and wisdom. We say that we understand that you cannot bring a baby into the world in a disinterested, disconnected or violent manner, and, oh, isn't birth—aren't babies—miraculous and wonderful?! And yet, we are quick to intervene in this natural process in numerous ways that upset the woman, the process and the newborn. We teach that "the experts" know best—rarely pausing long enough to remember that with all other mammals, the experts are the parents themselves. We all know that among other influences, the birth experience has an effect on how we parent and on the reactions, decisions and relations that we make as we begin to take care of our children in those early days. Andrea Frank Henkart is one of those people who understands the connection among pregnancy, birth, parenting and life. She knows that how we partner, and how we parent (just a switch of letters from partnering to parenting!), arises from a number of factors, and that when the majority of these are pleasant and positive, so too are our relationships with ourselves and with each other. She knows that how women birth, how they feel physically, emotionally, psychologically, nutritionally, sexually and spiritually during pregnancy and birth is important. She asks us to be mindful: positive support during pregnancy, birth and parenting is an essential key toward total health, joy and nonviolence in our world.

She understands the intricate patterns that are created—in the early moments, months and years of our lives that affect the rest of our lives.

In my own work, I see how the birth experience itself affects women and their infants for years. Early parenting becomes even more physically difficult and emotionally draining by the bruises (I refer to them as battle scars) that most women must heal after their "routine," "unremarkable" or "uneventful" deliveries. Technology-oriented birth and cesarean section are of grave concern to many of us in the childbirth movement. We all know that women are constantly subjected to unnecessary, unreliable and dangerous procedures, tests and surgery. As one example, recently, the National Citizens Research Group stated unequivocally that at least fifty percent of the cesareans that are performed are unnecessary (by my own observation, estimation and experience, that figure is far too conservative). Women were designed to have babies and to come through the experience safely and joyfully. Babies were designed to experience birth and to arrive alive, alert and ready for life. Generations of disempowered and drugged childbearing women, and incised and debilitated new mothers, create a society of drugged, disconnected and disoriented babies—whose first experiences on our earth ultimately leave us all exhausted and depressed. This sets the stage for difficulties which can be long-lasting; it is deeply distressing when we consider that with an opening of our hearts, a commitment toward genuine interpersonal caring and a willingness to trust, so much could be changed in so little time.

Andrea, thank you. Thank you for being one of the voices that makes sense in the raging cesarean seas. Thank you for creating a book that gives not only vital information but great opportunity for healing as well. You have blended your own personal experience and wisdom with that of others. I applaud your courage—fear turned inside out—in bringing together a group of visionaries and healers who speak up for wholeness, choice, respect and nature; they speak out against the current technological tides and implore us to think intuitively and intellectually. I am most impressed with the rainbow of authors you united who contributed to this work—strong, bold, gentle and accurate Truth-seekers/tellers. We are all connected in this world—how just one baby is born affects many people deeply. For that reason, as well as many others, we have an investment in one another's births; we must continue to educate the sleeping and the arrogant and the uneducated as to the horrendous complications of "birth-without-mothers"—deliveries with predominantly drugged, anesthetized or frightened (and therefore emotionally distanced) women. I found myself underlining, exclamation-pointing and considering anew so much of what you and your gifted partners in this endeavor have put forth. Indeed, although "the doctor" and the scientific/technocratic way (what Laura Shanley has dubbed the self-appointed "officialdom") are doing their best to control and monopolize birth and parenting, the women themselves and the loving parents of that infant are—and must be—the qualified contenders of those sacred and miraculous challenges.

Childbirth and parenting encompass power, strength, healing and joy. This book emphasizes that and much, much more. Andrea has given birth to this work, and has done it well. The words herein actually breathe—they inspire—and in that respect, the work itself is alive. I am honored to have had the privilege to read it. May it gently touch the minds and the hearts of those who read it, taking them swiftly to a personal place of knowing, and joining them in a connected space of "Yes!"

Foreword
Michel Odent, M.D.

On the very day when Andrea Frank Henkart asked me to write a foreword to *Trust Your Body! Trust Your Baby!* I received a phone call from my daughter. She wanted to tell me that her baby had just been born. She was thrilled about her baby boy, bursting to tell me what he was like: his shape, his movements, his weight (8 pounds), the color of his eyes, etc. . . . Just before I hung up, I asked her some specific questions about the delivery. She felt the first contractions at 7 P.M. and the baby was born at 7:55 P.M. Full stop.

There is a common point among women who have easy births. They "forget" to talk about it. It is only when my mother was in her late nineties that she answered my questions and gave me some details about my own birth. Up to that time I only heard her express what her feelings had been *after* the birth. The first contractions started at 10 P.M. and I was born at midnight (she was a 35-year-old first-time mother).

There are probably several reasons why such women are discreet about their deliveries. One reason is that when labor and delivery are intense and fast, it implies that the mother-to-be is really "on another planet." She has partly switched off the activity of her rational brain. Another reason is that giving birth, like making love, is seen as a private experience that isn't discussed. Also, an easy and fast birth implies that there were few people around to tell the story afterward, that is, there was nobody else other than an experienced and noninvasive midwife.

Thanks to such stories we are in a position to understand a paradox. Only women who have experienced difficulties and belong to the same generation can help and actually offer to help those who don't feel confident in their physiological potential. The lack of self-confidence is more and more common after several generations of medicalized birth.

Andrea is a typical example of a woman who has experienced difficulties when giving birth and who is able to understand the need for help from others.

I have a special interest in the background of women who can be classified as "childbirth reform activists." Their awareness and the energy they spend to help others always originates from well-defined personal experiences. One of my favorite stories is the biography of a little girl from North Dakota, Jody McLaughlin, who became the American editor of *The Compleat Mother*. When she was a girl living on her parents' farm near Bismarck, her father told her how to behave when a sow gives birth. He said, "Don't show yourself. Stay hidden. If the sow feels watched the delivery will be longer, more difficult, more dangerous; and, after the birth, she might have no interest in her babies. She might even become aggressive. So make yourself inconspicuous—but be aware of what is happening. Although the sow is the most competent mother imaginable, she might accidentally neglect or suffocate one of her eight or ten or more babies. If this happens, you should intervene discreetly and tactfully, only to protect the safety of the little pigs by moving them out of harm's way and returning them to suckle once the sow has again lain down on her side."

When this girl grew up, she had children of her own. To give birth, she went to a hospital and had to lie down on a table surrounded by experts who were telling her to push, or not to push, or to breathe in this way or that. She discovered that they knew nothing about birth, and she realized that it was thanks to her father and thanks to non-human mammals that she could trust her body and trust her baby.

Acknowledgments

It started as a dream, a thesis, a guidebook. Inspired by all the women who shared their births and their stories with me.

Supporting you while you brought life into this world was an honor. Watching as you birthed sons and daughters from your vaginas and your stomachs was a miracle. With each birth I wept. Your strength and your vulnerability touched me deeply. Your stories healed me as you healed yourselves. Thank you for sharing your most intimate woman experience with me.

I was supported by my dear friend and spiritual practitioner Reverend Ari Smith through all the ups and downs that life can bring. You are a bright star who shines down upon me whenever I am in need. I am blessed to know you.

I have been encouraged by my sisters in ways too numerous to mention. Suzanne Arms, Jeannine Parvati Baker, Esther Booth Zorn, Elizabeth Davis, Robbie Davis-Floyd, Gina Farber, Joan Flax-Clark, Judy Garland, Donna Germano, Lisa Gery, Robin Lim, Marilyn Milos, Ashley Storey and Nancy Wainer Cohen. Thank you for the richness you have added to my life.

To all the women who have touched my life: my family, my friends, my clients, my teachers and my midwives, I am forever grateful.

To Lynn Flint, Cathryn Lee and Dina Rubin at Greenwood Publishing Group; three voices at the end of the telephone umbilical cord. Thank you for your patience as I pushed this baby out my way.

A special thanks to my extended family, Bonnie and John Gray. Your unconditional love has been a guiding light throughout the years, your insight has been a blessing. I love you both.

And to Madame Francine Dierman Henkart, my mother-in-law. You effortlessly gave birth to five babies at home beginning in 1931. In 1946, you gave birth prematurely. You placed your tiny son in a doll carriage and kept him warm. You breastfed him on request and gave him love. No incubators, no tubes, no fear. Your strength, your dignity, your determination and your unconditional love have kept all fifty-one of your children, grandchildren and great grandchildren going strong. My hat is off to you, dear lady.

Lastly, I offer my heartfelt thanks to my best friend in the whole entire world, my incredible husband Reggie. Your love, support and patience are truly a gift of the Goddess.

TRUST YOUR BODY! TRUST YOUR BABY!

Chapter 1

Great Expectations
Andrea Frank Henkart

Andrea Frank Henkart has a Bachelor's Degree in Sociology from UCLA, two teaching credentials with an emphasis on alternative methods of education from UCLA Graduate Division, and a Master's Degree in Psychology from Sonoma State University. She holds a degree in Holistic Health from Heartwood Institute, and is a Certified Childbirth Educator and Certified Childbirth Assistant. Andrea was a Birth Management Consultant in private practice for over 10 years. Practicing in the United States, Mexico and Europe after studying advanced courses in yoga, massage, and midwifery, she provided counseling; prenatal massage and yoga; childbirth, health and parenting education; and birth assistance with an emphasis on cesarean prevention to pregnant couples. As co-founder and past president of the Marin County chapter of the International Cesarean Awareness Network, Ms. Henkart lectures and leads numerous workshops internationally on such issues as health, childbirth, parenting and personal growth. She is the author of The Cesarean Challenge *(1991).*

I was introduced to childbirth by a silent knife. It crept up on me when I least expected it. While pregnant with my first child, I did not plan for natural childbirth; I wanted a purebirth. Nancy Wainer Cohen and Lois Estner (1983) define purebirth as

> Birth that is completely free of medical intervention. Purebirth requires loving support, comfort and guidance from people who have positive energy to contribute to the birth environment. Where "natural" birth is a system designed and perpetuated by physicians as a medical event, purebirth is childbearing as an act of mother love, a way of thinking and feeling about birth

that allows us to take responsibility for the experience in whatever way we choose. (p. 120)

As an educator of holistic health and a student of spiritual midwifery, I was prepared to have my first child at home. I was strong,
healthy, determined and unaccepting of any other way of giving
birth. My midwife was a beautiful "earth-mother" from Santa Cruz,
California.

Because I was certified in massage therapy, nutritional counseling,
prenatal/postpartum yoga and rebirthing, my clients came to me
seeking a more holistic path. My viewpoint was somewhat limited,
as I was unwilling to talk to anyone who thought babies should be
born anywhere but at home. I was eating organic vegetarian cuisine,
walking two miles every day, meditating, diligently practicing yoga
and chanting and taking regular soaks in a hot tub heated to body
temperature. Everyone kept telling me that because I was in such
good shape, and because I was so "mellow" I would have no trouble
giving birth at home.

I had my first rude awakening when labor day arrived. It showed
up with a big gush of amniotic fluid waking me from a sound sleep.
Labor was hard and painful, yet I managed to get through it. I spent
many, many hours lying on my bed with my midwife, her assistant
and my husband by my side. I did finally dilate to ten centimeters
and earnestly began pushing my baby out. I remember suddenly feeling very fearful that I would rip open. Somewhere deep within myself I realized that as I gave birth to a child, I would have to give up
being a little girl myself. Motherhood meant responsibility that I was
not sure I was fully ready for. These thoughts were lost, however, as
the intensity of pushing a human being out of my vagina took over
my psyche and my body.

As the pain and intensity increased, something deep within my
soul told me I could not do this work. I still was not aware of this on
a conscious level. What I experienced consciously was uncertainty,
pain, fear and exhaustion. My daughter decided the timing was in-
appropriate for her and slid back inside me. My cervix closed down
to six centimeters and my midwife panicked!

A quick telephone call to her friend who was the head nurse at the
local community hospital prompted my midwife to suggest we go to
the hospital to see what was happening. By this time I was open to
anything. I was teetering between reality and other-world consciousness.

In retrospect, I realize that I should have been upright: walking, squatting, encouraged to stay grounded in my body. Homeopathic remedies administered at different points throughout my labor might have smoothed things along. I should have been prepared prenatally; I should have talked more prenatally, about life, my baby, anything and everything. But alas, that did not happen. So off to the hospital I went.

Disturbed by predators, a laboring animal in the wild will stop her birth process completely and find a safer location to birth. Like the wild animal, I shut down in response to the change in environment because of my intense fear of hospitals. As my fear level rose, my pain threshold lowered. My contractions became unbearably painful. The doctor suggested x-rays, Pitocin and a cesarean section in the event nothing else worked. He apparently was not very worried, suggested I wait it out, and literally offered me two hours in which to "perform."

The x-ray experience to me, the purist, was horrendous. How could they possibly take an x-ray of my unborn child and expose the two of us to an unnecessary amount of radiation? I believed those people had no morals whatsoever! The results of their penetrating, internal photographs showed that my pelvis was "small to normal," which in medical terms is not necessarily indicative of anything! The doctor was certain I could push my baby out vaginally with the assistance of an intravenous drip of Pitocin, and an external monitor emitting continual ultrasound right into my belly.

This was such a shock to me that I actually opted for a cesarean section! I had no idea what I was getting into. All I knew was that I wanted them to get my baby out of me with the least intervention possible. Somewhere along the way, I had lost my rational mind and assumed that major abdominal surgery was the least invasive.

When given a choice of an epidural or general anesthesia, I opted for the latter. Under no circumstances could I watch my belly be cut open and I did not want to participate in the hospital preliminaries.

Waking up in recovery was horrible. I didn't know what had hit me. I did not realize that it was morphine that hit me, or Demerol that was being put into my veins even as I tried to recover. I wanted to know whether I had given birth to a boy or a girl. I wanted to know whether my baby was alive, healthy, had all of her toes and fingers. Did she have any hair? Did she already hate me for starting her off on a life surrounded by hospital staff, drugs and insensitivity? The nurse assured me I was okay and walked out of the room. I was alone and scared and wanted my child.

When I awoke in my hospital room, my husband was standing right next to me holding our tiny (six pounds, seven ounces) daughter in his arms. She was beautiful. She was perfect. She held no grudges. I reached out to hold her but was instantly thwarted as pain tore through the core of my being. No one told me how much I would hurt *afterward*.

Those first few "daze" in the hospital were so different from anything I had experienced before. We were told our perfect little baby had neonatal jaundice. *Now* I know she did not have abnormal jaundice. Doctors and nurses often explain things to uninformed people in a very threatening manner. What really happened is that she was slightly yellow and had I nursed her continuously and held her in the sunshine through my hospital room window, she would have been fine within twenty-four to forty-eight hours. The hospital staff could not stand a no-intervention policy. They scared us into believing that if we did not intervene, it was *possible* our newborn could suffer brain damage and we would be held responsible.

Everything happened so fast. Because of fear, pain, confusion and lack of knowledge to decipher the lingo of the medical staff, we agreed to save the life of our baby, who was, as it turned out, in no real danger.

They wheeled in a plastic box with very bright lights attached to the top. Our baby was unswaddled from her warm blanket, her diaper was removed and they put a black, Halloween-type face mask over her tiny little eyes. She was then laid on her stomach in this enclosed case.

Two round circles were cut out on the front side of the box, so we could stick in our very sterilized and gloved hands to console our screaming newborn. Heaven forbid our germs which united to form this child and nourished her within my womb should come in contact with her on the outside of my womb! My husband and I stood there, each with one hand in the box, trying to get our sweet baby to know we were there to protect her from the evils of life. We were helpless. We were tired. We were scared. She remained in that box for hours, and she screamed the entire time. When we finally realized that she was too feisty to be sick, we insisted they stop their invasive treatment and let her out of that box.

We were no longer victims. In that moment of liberating our baby from the ridiculously bright light box, we liberated ourselves and found our own personal power. This was our baby, and we were going to have a say in anything they wanted to do to her in the name of prevention.

Once home from the hospital, I remember being in so much pain I could not believe one human being could suffer so much. I had never been very sick in my life, never had a broken bone or a cavity! At that time in my life, physical pain and I were not very well acquainted.

Mental anguish was the next stranger I met. I felt guilt and shame for not being able to push my baby out. I could not understand how I could have failed my husband, my child or myself.

My husband had wanted to see our first-born come out. He wanted to "catch" her as she made her entrance into this world. He had hoped to cut her umbilical cord as a rite of passage into fatherhood.

Lost in my own feelings of guilt, I was convinced my daughter would be damaged for life. She would grow up feeling abused, abandoned and unloved. She would wonder why I did not fight to birth her normally. I was sure that I had failed as a mother even before I started. I truly believed that I had failed at the basic test of life: womanhood. I could not be initiated into the club that billions of other women had participated in since the beginning of time. I was doomed. Yet, people around me insisted that I was behaving foolishly. I had to be thankful that my baby and I were alive. I needed to feel grateful that I had a healthy child. I had to stop being so silly and get on with my life.

Women who give birth by major abdominal surgery are often told to feel grateful, be happy and thank their lucky stars. The reality is that many women who give birth by major abdominal surgery often are overwhelmed by feelings of guilt and resentment. They feel victimized, angry, ripped off, sad, fearful and confused.

A few days after I came home from the hospital, I was mournfully sitting on my couch while my new baby slept peacefully in my arms. As my friend Bonnie walked in the door, I burst into tears and apologized to her for not having had a natural childbirth! I asked her whether she thought my daughter and I would ever have a good relationship. Bonnie took my hand in hers and gently said, "Andrea, both of my daughters were born by cesarean section." Knowing that her daughters were healthy and that she had a wonderful relationship with her girls gave me hope. Perhaps I did not fail.

Time passed, and I slowly adjusted to being a new mother. I surrendered to the process of total mothering. I nursed on request, our

infant slept in our bed, we carried her around and loved her unconditionally. I realized I had been foolish all along. Over the next couple of years, I had an annoying feeling tugging at me from the inside.
I never could really put my finger on it until I began therapy for
some childhood issues I wanted to process. Much to my surprise, my
cesarean anger came up all over again.

I heard about an organization called the Cesarean Prevention
Movement (CPM), currently known as the International Cesarean
Awareness Movement (ICAN). I excitedly called them up just to find
out what they were all about. After four years of swallowing feelings
I could not identify, I was actually talking to someone who completely understood! Evidently there were hundreds of women who
felt as I did, and there were meetings where I could talk to some of
those women. My husband and I listened as new mothers and fathers
came together and shared their birth stories. There were horror stories and there were success stories. These women knew how I felt.
They understood my obsession and my anger over my failed homebirth. The camaraderie was inspiring.

CPM sponsored an evening with Dr. Michel Odent. I had read his
book, *Birth Reborn* (1984), and was eager to hear what he had to
say about childbirth, cesarean prevention and vaginal birth after cesarean (VBAC, pronounced vee-back). Dr. Odent was inspiring. I
knew that my next birth experience would be different.

Pregnant with my second child, I was more than determined to have
a homebirth. I still believe that the most natural place for a child to be
born is at home. Hospitals are for people who are sick or have a disease. Medical technology can save lives; it can also screw up a perfectly
normal birth. Having a baby does not have to be a medical event.

We moved when I was five months pregnant with my second child.
Trying to find a midwife to assist me with my VBAC at home was a
difficult task. Doors were shutting in my face left and right. No one
wanted to help me; the politics were too risky. One midwife could
not get a doctor to back her up, another midwife could not risk her
reputation with a "high risk" homebirth, and still another midwife
did not have hospital privileges should the need to transport me to
the hospital arise.

I finally found myself in the office of two midwives who were willing to listen to my story. Because I had acted as vice president for the
Los Angeles chapter of the Cesarean Prevention Movement for a
short time and founded the Marin County chapter, these midwives
knew I was determined, yet they still hesitated.

My husband and I sat in their office and literally begged them to support us through our process of childbirth at home. I remember asking them to look closely at the work they do. Isn't midwifery about women supporting women? Historically, many midwives risked their lives to assist women in labor. Midwives were hanged for practicing witchcraft, yet they did not give up. Could these modern day midwives just turn their back on a sister in need?

With tears in their eyes, they lovingly agreed to work with us, providing we found our own doctor who would act as back-up should a hospital transport become necessary. After every doctor in the immediate area refused to back up a home VBAC because it was "too risky" or "too dangerous" or they could not risk their own reputation among their colleagues, my midwives decided should I need to go to the hospital, we would just leave the county and drive to the city. I assured them I would not need a hospital for the birth of my child.

Once again, labor day came, bringing with it excitement and joy. During early labor, I walked around my neighborhood, swam a few laps in our swimming pool and waited with anticipation. My first strong contraction literally knocked the wind out of me. I kept walking, knowing that upright movement was the best thing for this stage of labor. But the contractions kept getting stronger and more painful. This was a pain I could not come to grips with. It was a pain that was rocking me from the very core of my being, like an earthquake shaking Mother Nature from the center of the Earth.

Labor can bring a woman face to face with every fear she has ever known. This happens on a subconscious level and can take over with no warning sign at all. I was lost in fear as the pain of my contractions racked my body. I was out of control, and neither my midwives, my husband nor God could help me now. I felt like I was spiraling downward into the sea of Hell.

How is it that millions of women give birth easily and effortlessly? Many women never take a childbirth class or read a book on birth. Yet there I was, highly educated, well informed, dedicated to homebirth, yet still unable to give birth naturally. "Maybe you need to rest, let's take you to the hospital. They'll give you something to relax you," my midwife said trying to sound convincing.

I was taken to a nearby hospital in the city where the labor and delivery nurses were eagerly awaiting "the VBAC Lady." "You can do it," they cried. "You're gonna push this baby right out of your vagina, we just know it," they urged. With big smiles full of hope, the nurses hooked me up to numerous machines. When the blood pressure cuff malfunctioned and the external fetal monitor stopped working and the intravenous drip popped out of my veins, I knew I was in trouble.

The anesthesiologist confidently concluded, "This epidural will numb you so that you can sleep. Once you are rested you can begin to labor again." With false hope I allowed them to stick a catheter into my spinal column and inject a strong medication to help me relax. They insisted any medication they administered would not pass into my womb. How is it that cigarette smoke, alcohol and every bite of food eaten by a pregnant woman affects the health and well-being of her unborn child, yet the strong medication used by doctors to numb pain, induce labor or "take the edge off" labor does not hurt the baby?

Fifty minutes into the epidural anesthetic, I was in pain again. The Pitocin that was given to me to bring on contractions was stronger than the medication given to numb the pain from those contractions. The anesthesiologist said that it was impossible for me to be in pain so soon. The medication was set to ease up after approximately two hours. Not only was I experiencing excruciating pain, I was also being called a liar. "The medication could not be wearing off so quick," he responded in an angry tone.

My midwife was finally so distraught at the way I was declining in spirit and frustrated at the malfunctioning machines surrounding me, she stopped the Pitocin and yanked the needles out of my arm. After screaming for two hours that the pain induced by the medication was beyond human tolerance, I was grateful someone had finally stopped the madness.

Left alone in the room, I was scared and exhausted. The doctors and nurses secretly discussed my "case" with my midwives and my husband outside my room. The irony was that I could hear them through the closed door. I screamed out for them to talk *to* me, not *about* me behind my back. The doctors were not interested in discussing anything with me, as doctors often believe that a woman in labor cannot make any rational decisions for herself. I was extremely rational and was determined to participate in all decisions made about me.

The next anesthesiologist on duty suggested a cesarean section. "No sense torturing yourself like this, my dear," he said with authority. He was right. This was torture. I demanded a cesarean, and the doctors refused! "You can have the vaginal birth you hoped for," cheered the doctors and nurses. Still no one was listening to me. Like a pain-ridden cancer victim requesting the right to die, I was requesting a cesarean section to end my own pain. This was my body, my baby and my birth.

Looking back, I can remember two more significant events that transpired during that long, painful labor in the hospital. As my cervix was desperately trying to dilate, a resident doctor came in to examine me. By that time I had lost count of how many different sets of hands had measured my cervical dilation. As the doctor was checking me, she excitedly reported I had dilated to nine centimeters. With ten centimeters being the goal, she suggested they unhook all the machinery and let me push my baby out. I remember my midwife and I crying for joy. I was almost there! I had finally made it! My husband had been taking a nap after being at my side for the last forty hours. Someone excitedly rushed off to awaken him with the good news.

The doctor on duty came in to check me again before "allowing" me to birth my child. Upon his inspection, he was sorry to say that the other doctor had made a mistake and I was "only" four centimeters dilated. *She made a mistake.* "Carry on," the doctor suggested; "these things happen." My midwife held me in her arms as we both cried.

At some point, Bonnie, who had been invited to the birth, came into the labor and delivery room where I had been hooked up to machines for hours. I felt like Frankenstein's monster, lying there like somebody's laboratory experiment. She stood over my bed, holding my hand with a look of pity and sadness in her eyes. "How are you *really?*" she lovingly inquired.

Bonnie had just recently had a VBAC in the hospital, so I asked her what it was like to push a baby out of her body. She related her own personal experience to me, telling me it hurt but was worth it. I remember telling her that I honestly did not believe that my body could do it. Intuitively, I believed that something inside me was blocking me from allowing my baby to enter the world vaginally.

As they wheeled me into the operating room, the anesthesiologist assured me that the epidural anesthesia would be effective during surgery and that I should not experience any pain. He did say, however, that I might experience a sensation of tugging and pulling.

After I was strapped down and prepped for surgery an appropriate dose of medication was injected into my body. The anesthesiologist then took a pin and began to lightly prick my legs and belly to make sure I was appropriately numbed for the operation. I immediately informed him that I could feel the pin and that it hurt! He said that was impossible. Confused, exhausted and angry, my husband told the doctor that I was not in the habit of telling lies. The doctor refused to listen to him and assured the surgeons that I was ready to be cut.

With the first cut came a searing pain in my gut. I wanted to die. I do not remember opening my mouth and screaming, but later the nurses told me they heard my screams on the entire floor. My mind was reeling as my body kept screaming with pain. "Stop the torture; stop the torture." One of the surgeons likened it to a nineteenth century surgery. She said she had never seen anything like that before.

The anesthesiologist should have given me a general anesthetic to put me to sleep, but he was afraid I would aspirate on the water I had sipped during labor. With all the technology hospitals offer, there must be a drug or a machine that can prevent a patient from vomiting during labor. Instead, the brilliantly trained medical man injected me with a shot of Valium to relax me. Valium did not relax me, but caused my unborn child to experience distress. When that did not work, he injected a drug called ketamine into my veins. Ketamine is often used by veterinarians, rarely by medical doctors. The drug is a hallucinogen, which caused me to go on a psychedelic trip.

As I bounced off the pink puffy walls of my uterus, I was lost in the folds of skin and could not find my way out. I was being tickled by blood vessels and veins that were floating by me, as I kept sinking further and further into the folds of my skin. I became claustrophobic and wanted out. "Help me, save me," I kept shouting. My husband was steadfast and strong by my side throughout the entire ordeal. But the moment he heard me say, "It still hurts," with a very other-worldly, euphoric laugh, he could no longer bear my pain.

They pulled a strong, healthy, eight pound, fourteen ounce boy out of my womb before piecing me back together and sewing me up. The surgeon discovered that some of the pain I experienced during labor was due to incorrect placement of my bladder when they put it back after the first cesarean. I never knew it was out of place!

I woke up in my room late that night and was determined to get out of that hospital as soon as possible. I knew exactly what I had to do to expedite my recovery so I could go home. To the surprise of the night nurse, I attempted to walk immediately. I attempted polarity therapy by massaging my shins as much as I could to facilitate the famous passing of gas after abdominal surgery. I kept my baby next to me and nursed him as much as possible so that my uterus would continue to contract. This would expedite my internal physical healing, while providing nourishment to my baby.

The anesthesiologist came to visit me in my room the next morning. He apologized for my "unfortunate experience." He seemed to be sweet-talking me, suggesting I not sue him and his staff. He had no logical explanation for what happened to me during labor or delivery. He said they did all they could. I have told my story to many obstetricians and surgeons, who have all unanimously agreed that I should have been given general anesthesia. Perhaps my doctors could have done more after all.

When the nurse suggested my newborn son had skin that was looking a little yellow, I began immediate and continual breast-feeding. No one was going to convince me my child had jaundice this time, and I was not going to put this baby into a light box. I telephoned my pediatrician for advice. He suggested I "wait it out" and told the resident pediatrician on duty to leave us alone!

Three days later, I was ready to go home. I told the doctor on call that I wanted to be released. She suggested I stay a few more days. Had I been vacationing in a luxurious hotel, I might have considered staying. However, I was in a hospital and I wanted to go home! I told her I was aware of my rights as a patient, and that I could check myself out against medical advice. Without hesitation, the doctor decided I could be paroled and signed my release papers. I was home free.

Recovery at home was easier the second time around. I was more comfortable at home, and my son was now surrounded by the love of his father and big sister. I was grateful to be in my own environment and ready to begin the healing process of cesarean birth all over again.

My involvement with the Marin County chapter of the Cesarean Prevention Movement became stronger. I started making telephone calls from my bed as I continued to recuperate at home. I lined up speakers for our monthly meetings and found other women who wanted to share their cesarean birth stories.

Our meetings grew, and our sudden popularity caused a storm in the collective obstetric consciousness. Doctors were becoming angry when their patients told them they wanted VBACs and were active members of CPM. Over a three year period, our chapter volunteers educated and informed hundreds of women about their choices and their rights in childbirth.

As I listened to the stories of other women, I began to heal from my own trauma. I told my own story over and over and was soon invited to speak at various events and conferences. What I encountered were hundreds of women who had simple, basic questions about childbirth and cesarean prevention. I could not understand why they were not getting this information from their doctors or childbirth educators.

Pregnant women must take personal responsibility in the planning of their pregnancy, labor and delivery. Expectant parents must educate themselves about the physical and psychological processes of childbirth. Becoming aware of hospital or birth center policies and regulations give the laboring woman the power and the knowledge to make conscious choices. Women must reconsider the medically oriented way they give birth. We must reclaim the normal, natural process of giving birth, and allow each child to experience his or her own unique entrance into this life.

Revel in the beauty that is pregnancy, body growing within body. Surrender to the tumultuous joy that is childbirth. Prepare for the death of that part of the soul that has not yet given life to this baby and open to the birth of the emerging mother. Allow the miracle of childbirth to carry you through your own individual ride into parenthood. Leave fear behind as you celebrate the birth of a human being. Listen to your deep inner voice. Trust your body! Trust your baby!

Chapter 2

On the Cutting Edge
Andrea Frank Henkart

When a woman goes into labor, especially with a first birth, a typical scenario runs something like this: contractions begin, the bag of water may break, there is great excitement in the air. She tells her partner, who also becomes nervous and excited. The big day is finally here! She moves around a little to see if these pains are the real thing, and eventually makes that first phone call to her doctor. The doctor tells her to "come on down."

After arriving at the hospital and checking in, the excited couple begin to fix up the room. Video camera here, tape recorder there. Her slippers, gown and robe are all neatly hung in the tiny closet of the birthing room. This room is supposed to look just like their bedroom, but suddenly the couple realizes this is not as comfortable or inviting as home. Trying to make the best of the situation, they begin to walk around the room when the nurse walks in. The laboring woman changes into a hospital gown after she is told that the nightshirt she planned on laboring in might get messy. With contractions increasing in strength, she excitedly gets on the bed to be checked. Feeling fairly confident that things are progressing quickly (after all, she went to childbirth classes, read a few books, and took prenatal aerobics while pregnant), her world begins to close in on her when she is told, "You're *only* two centimeters dilated; sit back and relax, honey, because you have a long way to go."

After what seem like endless vaginal examinations to determine how many centimeters she has dilated, and many hours later, the woman becomes exhausted. Her morale starts to fade and the fear that something may be wrong with her baby slowly begins to invade her thoughts. The occasional use of the external fetal monitor now becomes continuous. Her exhaustion is mounting and she becomes dehydrated from lack of food or liquids. To give her more energy, intravenous fluid is inserted into her vein while she lies flat on her back on the bed. Now that she realizes that she is hooked up and immobile, the remainder of her faith is depleted. Next comes Pitocin to stimulate labor, an epidural to numb her from pain, more fear, more unconscious feelings of failure, a small dip in heart tones for the baby, and the woman in labor who planned a simple, non-invasive birth may now be on her way to a cesarean section.

This story has been written to illustrate a common phenomenon in childbirth, namely, the cesarean section operation. As a certified childbirth assistant for over ten years, and co-founder and past president of the Marin County chapter of the International Cesarean Awareness Network, I am deeply concerned about this growing problem. Women have told me that their doctors often suggest that they "allow" them to break the bag of water to "speed things up." Their doctors are known to say, "Let's just give you a *little* Pitocin to get 'things' going." Women have told me over and over again how these scenarios cause them to shut down, become fearful and doubt themselves and the well-being of their unborn child. I have heard women state again and again how these scenarios have led them to have a cesarean section, or a surgical-vaginal birth resulting from overuse of episiotomy and gadgets such as forceps, vacuum extraction and fetal monitors.

Some doctors may unconsciously take advantage of the vulnerability of a woman in labor. The words they use can be unconsciously interpreted by a laboring woman as threatening or negative. According to my client Linda, when her obstetrician confirmed that she was pregnant, he also told her she might need a cesarean section if she got too big. Over the years, I have heard so many doctors tell pregnant women that they have an untested uterus and therefore may have trouble, or that they have a small to normal pelvis. According to Cohen (personal communication, 1994), these statements often have no foundation, in addition to the fact that they program a pregnant woman with negative ideas and fears.

Originally, cesarean sections were performed to remove the fetus from a dead mother. Flamm (1990, p. 18) found, "At times this surgery was done soon after the mother's death in an attempt to save the baby. Later the operation was performed on living women but only when it was absolutely impossible for the baby to be born vaginally." He goes on to say, "It should be stressed that the cesarean operation was developed as a radical intervention to assist the rare woman who was physically incapable of giving birth naturally." A report by Harris in 1879 showed that cesarean sections had been performed on sixteen dwarfs because of pelvic deformity. Eleven of the sixteen women died from the operation.

The first cesarean documented in the United States (Speert, 1980) was performed by Doctor John Richmond in Newton, Ohio, in April 1827. A 1916 article by E. B. Cragin showed that less than one percent of women had cesarean sections to deliver their babies. Today, cesarean section is the most common major surgical operation performed in our country and the most frequently performed unnecessary surgery (Gabay and Wolfe, 1994). Our national cesarean rate is now 22.6 percent (966,000 cesarean births in 1992). In *Unnecessary Cesarean Sections: Curing a National Epidemic* (1994), Gabay and Wolfe say

> Today, nearly one in four women passing through the doors of a labor and delivery suite will undergo major abdominal surgery. Many of these operations, which pose a greater risk of maternal complications and even death than vaginal delivery, are medically unnecessary. It is unconscionable that every day unnecessary cesarean surgery is performed on thousands of women, squandering valuable millions of health care dollars, while almost forty million Americans lack basic health insurance.

The United States Department of Health and Human Services (1990) found that cesarean sections are the most common surgical operation performed in hospitals, surpassing procedures such as tonsillectomies, hysterectomies, hernia repair and gall bladder removal.

Dr. Edward Quilligan, Professor Emeritus, University of California at Irvine and Co-Editor-in-Chief of the *American Journal of Obstetrics and Gynecology* has said the proper range of cesarean rates, if the operation is performed only when medically necessary, is between 7.8 percent and 17.5 percent (1983). Sandmire (1993) found documented cases of hospitals that serve large numbers of women with high-risk pregnancies that have achieved cesarean section rates far lower than 17.8 percent without increased perinatal mortality or morbidity. Based on numerous studies, Gabay and Wolfe estimate the optimal national and state cesarean section rate should be approximately twelve percent.

In their book *Unnecessary Cesarean Sections: Curing a National Epidemic* (1994), Gabay and Wolfe list the one hundred and six hospitals with the highest cesarean rates nationwide, with low rates ranging from thirty-seven percent up to the highest rate of 63.7 percent. If the local hospital in a woman's community has a high section rate she may automatically be at a higher risk for a cesarean, unless she is willing to drive miles to another hospital with lower cesarean statistics, or chooses to have a home birth.

Despite the increase in the number of cesarean sections performed, the United States continues to have one of the highest infant mortality rates among industrialized nations (*Health United States*, 1990). The United States infant and maternal death rates are higher than in over a dozen other developed nations where cesarean rates are lower and vaginal births after previous cesareans are the norm, not the exception.

The overuse of the cesarean section operation has created an image of risk-free, pain-free childbirth. Doctors and pregnant women often forget that a cesarean section *is* major abdominal surgery. While few types of surgery pose absolutely no risk whatsoever, birth by cesarean is a safer alternative for a baby who could be injured, or a woman who would otherwise die in labor. However, there are inherent risks and complications in giving birth by major abdominal surgery. Gabay and Wolfe (1994) cite negative psychological and emotional impacts, (possible) higher rate of infertility, infection, excessive bleeding requiring a transfusion, injuries to surrounding organs, abnormal blood clotting and maternal death (p. 20).

Technically, cesarean section is considered to be a life-saving operation. While leading seminars and workshops on cesarean awareness and prevention, I have heard hundreds of women say that their cesarean section saved their life and the life of their baby. However, an eleven year study by Evard and Gold (1977) found that the rate of death from cesarean section was twenty-six times higher than the rate of death from vaginal delivery. Women of childbearing age need to be cautioned! Once used as a method to save the fetus of a dead mother, childbirth by major abdominal surgery is often considered a "cure-all" to any problem that develops during labor.

Petitti, et al. (1982) also compared the cesarean mortality rate with that of vaginal birth. They concluded that the risk of maternal death due to cesarean birth was two to four times greater than the risk associated with vaginal delivery. Gabay and Wolfe (1994) agree. They say, "Even healthy women undergoing elective repeat cesareans (as opposed to those who need emergency c-sections) may face an increase of as high as fourfold in the likelihood of death during delivery, compared to those undergoing vaginal delivery."

During a cesarean operation, the baby is also at risk. Malloy, et al. (1991) found that cesarean sections are used commonly to deliver babies weighing under three pounds. The study was specifically designed to determine whether cesarean sections would produce better outcomes for these babies. They found that cesarean sections *did not* produce healthier babies.

A cesarean section does not guarantee a perfect baby. More and more women are pressuring their doctors to do whatever they can to deliver a flawless baby, and the doctors are obliging by performing cesarean sections. Many women falsely believe that by exposing themselves to the risks of major abdominal surgery they are guaranteed a healthier, more "perfect" baby. The most obvious example of harm caused by surgical delivery is iatrogenic prematurity, or doctor-caused prematurity. This happens when the baby is born too soon: in other words, when the due date is calculated incorrectly by the doctor. Lung problems found more frequently in babies born by cesarean section (respiratory distress syndrome and hyaline membrane disease) can be potentially fatal.

A baby born vaginally often has a squashed appearance after being squeezed through the birth canal. By contrast, a cesarean born baby has a smooth, round head. Yet it is the cesarean baby who needs more time to adjust after her sudden entrance into the world, because she has missed the process that stimulates her circulation and allows amniotic fluid to be squeezed from the depths of her mature lungs as she passes through the birth canal.

In personal conversations, three obstetricians who wish to remain anonymous (1994) reported horror stories of colleagues accidentally amputating fingers from a newborn's hand, or accidentally breaking bones while surgically removing the infant. "You know, these things happen," said one doctor matter-of-factly.

Susan came to me for labor support during her second pregnancy. She shared her own horror story. Early one Friday morning, Susan arrived at the hospital in early labor for the birth of her first child. Standard procedure in her hospital required that all women in labor be monitored. This included machines and tubes hooked up to Susan's unsuspecting body. Once bedridden and unable to move with ease, unable to walk around during labor to bring her baby farther down into her pelvis, and terrified of the dehumanizing experience, Susan was left in her hospital room to labor alone. She remembers the nurse saying, "You'll be fine, honey," and then walking out the door. Susan was frightened, and her contractions caused pain that she could not deal with while forced to lie down on a hard hospital bed.

It was late Friday night when her doctor came in to check her. Susan remembers he jokingly remarked that he had to celebrate his son's birthday the next day, so she better "hurry up!" After hours of minimal dilation, the doctor was concerned. He found no apparent fetal distress but told Susan she wasn't progressing as well as he had hoped. Among many obstetricians, there is a typical (unstated) standard for dilation, which is approximately one centimeter per hour. According to many obstetricians and midwives I have spoken to, first births are commonly known to take longer. However, Susan's doctor decided she needed a cesarean section.

In the very early hours of Saturday morning, the well-respected, caring doctor Susan hired to help deliver her baby was now cutting through layers of skin, fat, fascia, muscle, and internal organs, and finally into her uterus. His hand slipped ever so slightly, and this well-respected, caring doctor cut a huge gash into the right cheek of the baby still in utero. Susan's baby required plastic surgery to repair the "accident."

Susan decided to give birth to her second child at home. Her midwives were patient and reassuring while she labored for twenty-two hours. Susan reached down and ecstatically pulled her own child from her body. He was intact and healthy, weighing in at nine pounds, twelve ounces!

According to the Consumer Advocates for the Legalization of Midwives (CALM) in the state of California (1994), planned home-births with trained midwives in attendance are often as safe or safer than hospital births for most pregnancies. CALM also found that the five countries with the lowest infant mortality rates (Japan, Finland, Sweden, Norway and Denmark) utilize midwives as primary health care providers in over seventy percent of births.

According to Flamm (1990), the American College of Obstetrics and Gynecology (ACOG) is the largest organization of obstetricians and gynecologists in the world. In October 1988, ACOG revised its outdated philosophy of "once a cesarean, always a cesarean." ACOG's guidelines recommend that, in the absence of medical complications of pregnancy, all women with previous cesarean sections should be encouraged to attempt a VBAC. Despite this recommendation, the most common reason physicians cited for performing cesareans in 1991 was that the woman had undergone a previous cesarean section. Approximately 338,000 of the 966,000 cesareans performed in 1991 that resulted in live births were repeat cesareans (Gabay and Wolfe, 1994).

While some women are encouraged by their obstetricians to have a VBAC, some doctors are also telling them about the risks and dangers of the "procedure" so that fear of everything from complications, to pain, to uterine rupture, to infant death causes these women to opt for a repeat cesarean, which in fact has many more inherent dangers, side effects, and possible complications. Required by legal mandates and malpractice policies, doctors must inform their patients of the worst possible scenarios. They should also be required to soften their presentations.

In her book *Open Season* (1991), Nancy Wainer Cohen writes about Dr. Gerald Bullock, who says that he can guarantee a failed VBAC (1987). His advice includes:

> Doctors: . . . be noncommittal enough in the early interviews: the issues won't come up again until later in the pregnancy. It is the rare patient indeed who has the presence of mind and strength of conviction to change doctors late in pregnancy. During the pregnancy, be sure to add to the mystique of the previous cesarean by ordering several ultrasounds and suggesting an amniocentesis, so the mother will understand how different and potentially dangerous her situation is. Never mind informing her that the risk of amniocentesis is higher to the baby than the risk of VBAC. . . .
>
> If by chance the mother hears about cesarean prevention classes or VBAC group meetings, tell her they are a bunch of crazy radicals who have only their own crosses to burn and do not have her best interests in mind. . . .
>
> Tell them that the baby must . . . not weigh more than whatever is your own limit (never mind that your guess at the weight is often as much as two pounds off). . . . Make her understand that she will be laboring against a deadline. If you are not successful in getting the patient to consent to a repeat cesarean . . . early in labor, do not despair; all is not lost. There are several ways still in which you can get her to give up the notion of

VBAC. Make sure she remembers what a high-risk patient she is, and keep an ever constant vigil for "catastrophe." . . . Don't give in to the frivolous request to ambulate . . . she must therefore be confined to bed from the time of arrival to the time of delivery. . . . Be kind and considerate, and apologize for not being able to allow her more flexibility. . . . Say things like, "Of course, your baby's safety is our primary concern." . . .

When the patient arrives early in labor, look at her critically and say something like, "Do you really think that you are going to have that big thing from below?" . . . A note from anesthesiologists: Be sure that you come in fairly early to do your "routine preoperative history review." If you do it right, you can leave the impression that almost all VBAC mothers eventually go ahead with a repeat cesarean. . . . Explain what will happen "while" she has her cesarean, not "if" she has it. . . . Finally [for other staff members standing outside the door], you might say something like "Is that blood ready? Get it stat! What if she ruptures?" (p. 314)

Previously, cesarean sections were performed by utilizing a vertical incision, or the "classical cesarean delivery." In 1981, the U.S. Department of Health and Human Services indicated that modern obstetricians should use "the bikini cut," which is a small, horizontal incision across the lower part of the uterus, also known as a low transverse incision. This type of incision sharply reduces the chance of uterine rupture (Gabay and Wolfe, 1994). I heard one doctor say, "Your bikini cut is certainly less offensive to look at. I did a pretty good job." His patient replied, "Yes, but I know it's there and *that's* what matters."

According to Flamm (1990), uterine rupture is infrequent. It occurs in approximately less than half of one percent and is rarely cause for concern; recovery is usually normal and surgery is rarely necessary. Uteruses do not explode! Flamm goes on to say that this organ can stretch to enormous proportions to encompass the cord, placenta, large amounts of fluid, and the baby. Women undergoing a trial of labor for vaginal birth after a previous cesarean and women undergoing elective repeat cesareans have the same chance of uterine rupture, which is close to nil. Through numerous studies, Gabay and Wolfe (1994, p. 27) show that "the catastrophic rupture of the uterus feared by obstetricians is an extremely rare event." Cohen (1991) says, "The issue of uterine rupture is a non-issue" (p. 310).

A major issue in the increased rate of births by major abdominal surgery, however, is directly related to the cost of the operation. Throughout my experience as a childbirth assistant, I have been told by labor and delivery nurses that more cesarean operations are performed on certain days of the week, and before long weekends or major holidays, and that cesareans bring more money to the doctors and the hospitals. Gabay and Wolfe (1994) claim doctors receive up to twenty to forty percent more for performing a cesarean section. They also state, "We estimate that 473,000 of the 966,000 cesareans performed in 1991 (49.0 percent) were unnecessary, costing American society more than $1.3 billion." The Health Insurance Association of America (1992) has shown that the estimated physician fees for cesarean delivery are almost double the fees for vaginal delivery, and the extra days spent in the hospital after birth by major abdominal surgery roughly double hospital revenues for cesarean sections. Dr. Richard Schwartz (1991), president of ACOG estimated that a one percent drop in the national cesarean rate would save $115 million dollars annually. The amount of money saved could be used in AIDS research, to care for low birth weight and drug-addicted babies, to improve our schools, or for any number of health and social issues facing our culture.

There are medical indications which warrant a cesarean section, and, when a cesarean section is necessary, it can save the life of both mother and baby. Transverse lie, that is, when the baby is lying across the mother's abdomen horizontally as labor begins, is cause for a cesarean section. Unless the baby rotates itself while the mother is in labor, a baby cannot possibly pass through the vagina in this position. This "problem" occurs in only approximately two to three births out of one hundred (Flamm, 1990).

Placental problems which can cause hemorrhage may warrant emergency cesarean sections. Several studies (Flamm, 1990; Gaskin, 1990) show that placenta abruption, a premature separation of the placenta from the uterine wall before the baby is born, and placenta previa, when the placenta or the "afterbirth" blocks the birth canal occur only once in every two hundred births.

Four of the leading reasons doctors perform cesarean sections are: previous cesarean, breech position, fetal distress and dystocia. *Morbidity and Mortality Weekly* (1993) reported six out of seven cesareans (86.3 percent) were done for one of these clinical reasons in 1991 alone. Numerous studies have proven that the over-diagnosis and misdiagnosis of these "problems" have led to hundreds of thousands of unnecessary cesarean sections (Gabay and Wolfe, 1994).

Transverse and breech (head-up position) babies can often be "turned." This process is known as external version. A highly specific maneuver, this attempt to turn the baby into a vertex position should only be done by a skilled practitioner. However, Kitzinger (1990) says that many doctors nowadays do not know how to perform external version, preferring to deliver any baby in a "bad" position by cesarean section. Contrary to this preference, an English doctor told me most British and European obstetricians deliver breech babies vaginally, and in Holland many of the breech babies are born at home with the assistance of a midwife (W. Claire, M.D., 1994, personal communication). As babies move around in early pregnancy, a breech position is not uncommon. Approximately two thirds turn to a vertex presentation spontaneously, which leaves just three to four percent of babies in the breech position at delivery time (Gabay and Wolfe, 1994).

Some mothers are able to massage their babies into the vertex position by themselves; others have reported success using other methods such as herbs, homeopathic remedies, acupuncture, acupressure, chiropractic adjustments, visualization techniques and specific exercises.

The postural tilt is an exercise used to tip the baby up out of your pelvis. You must get into a knee-chest position on your front with your head on the floor and your hips as high as possible. Try leaning over a stack of pillows or a bean bag chair. To do the pelvic tilt, lie on your back and elevate your hips twelve inches off the ground using pillows for support. Keep your knees bent, your feet flat on the floor and your head flat on the ground. Choose whichever position is more comfortable, and remain in this position for fifteen minutes three times each day. Concentrate on relaxing your body completely and visualize your baby turning. Some babies will do a somersault even after thirty seven weeks (Kitzinger, 1990). If the baby does turn, be sure to walk around for one or two hours to keep the head down. Once the baby has rotated and stays in the preferred position, discontinue this exercise. While some babies will go right back into the breech position, Kitzinger (1990) says "seven times out of ten, external version at 37 to 39 weeks is successful." If your baby decides to remain in a breech position, watch birth videos that show babies born buttocks or feet first, read books that show photographs of breech births, and learn about body positioning during labor and delivery to dispel any fear you may have and to prepare for a joyous birth.

According to Flamm, *true* fetal distress, which has a one to five chance of occurrence every one hundred births, is usually caused by cord compression and diagnosed by late deceleration in fetal heart tones. He goes on to show that another medical emergency, prolapsed umbilical cord, that is, a cord that comes out of the cervix or vagina before or with the baby's head, occurs in only one out of every one hundred births.

Dystocia is a "catch-all" diagnosis for the abnormal progression of labor, including: prolonged labor, uterine inertia, arrest of active labor, prolonged second stage and cephalopelvic disproportion (CPD), when the baby's head appears too large to pass through the pelvis. The decision to perform a cesarean section for dystocia is not always straightforward. In 1991, dystocia accounted for 30.4 percent of all cesareans performed (*Morbidity and Mortality Weekly Report*, 1993). How labor is managed can have a dramatic effect on the cesarean section rate for this "problem." Gabay and Wolfe (1994) provide several studies that show how diagnosis and use of cesarean for dystocia vary widely according to geographic regions, hospitals and physicians. They also mention the "obstetrician impatience factor" in management of labor. Additional comments include, "This 'impatience factor' has been found in studies demonstrating that cesarean sections are performed more frequently in the evening or in cases where there are fewer obstetricians to share round-the-clock availability for labor and delivery."

Unless an epidemic of deformed pelvic bones has occurred, it is doubtful that women have lost the ability to give birth naturally. While I have shown that one in every four women has a cesarean section, many studies show that these same women do not have cesareans which are medically necessary. One in four women *does not* have an emergency cesarean! Therefore, according to these statistics, the unnecessary rise in the number of cesarean sections in America is not related to those cesareans that are deemed medically necessary.

While many non-emergency cesarean sections are necessary and life saving, a necessary cesarean does not always mean that the situation is an emergency. A placenta previa can be detected before it reaches an emergency state. A woman with a small placental abruption can be sectioned on a non-emergency basis. A maternal drug abuser unable to labor for numerous reasons may also need a non-emergency cesarean section.

Holly is a registered nurse who has worked in labor and delivery at a hospital in California for five years. She told me,

> The difference between a normal cesarean section and an emergency basically have to do with the anesthesia administered. There usually is no time for a spinal or an epidural to be administered, so a general anesthesia must be used. The preparation in getting the woman ready goes *really* fast, and the surgeon gets the baby out much quicker. We are talking life-saving here. The most common sections are done because the doctor thinks there is nothing left to do. At that point the women are so worn out, they agree with anything. It's funny, but so many women leave the hospital believing that their cesarean was an emergency, when it really wasn't. Some of the doctors make the patient feel like it is an emergency at the time, but it's rarely really an emergency. The doctor just wants to hurry up. As a nurse, I'm an employee of the hospital. There isn't a lot I can do about any of this if I want to keep my job.

Currently, birth in our country is seen as a disease and *not* the miracle that it is. Birthing normally is our God-given right as women on this earth. It appears the technology that in fact saves many mothers and babies is the very technology that is robbing us of our right to birth.

According to Esther Booth Zorn (1990), founder of the International Cesarean Awareness Network (ICAN), an international, nonprofit organization with over eighty chapters nationwide, "Natural Childbirth is in more trouble now than it was eight to ten years ago. It is being redefined by many as meaning whenever the baby emerges from the vagina" (p. 1). In her article in the *Clarion*, the newspaper distributed quarterly by ICAN, Zorn goes on to say, "Keeping a good distance from truly experiencing something while absolving oneself of any responsibility sits well with the present generation of birthing women. The push is on to promote natural birth on medical terms and women are buying it" (p. 1).

Chapter 3

Ritual in the Hospital:
Giving Birth the American Way

Robbie E. Davis-Floyd

Robbie E. Davis-Floyd is a Cultural Anthropologist specializing in medical and symbolic anthropology, gender studies, the anthropology of reproduction and futures research. She received her Ph.D. from the University of Texas at Austin, where she teaches anthropology and holds the position of Research Fellow. For the past ten years she has been conducting research on ritual, technology and childbirth in the United States. Articles she has written on this subject have appeared in various edited books and academic journals, including Social Science and Medicine, *the* Medical Anthropology Quarterly, Knowledge and Society *and the* Pre- and Perinatal Psychology Journal. *The mother of two children, Dr. Davis-Floyd is the author of* Birth as an American Rite of Passage. *She recently completed the updating and expansion of Brigitte Jordan's landmark book* Birth in Four Cultures, *and, with Carolyn Sargent, is co-editing a collection of anthropological articles on* Childbirth and Authoritative Knowledge: Cross-Cultural Perspectives. *She lectures around the country on ritual and technology in American birth, the power of ritual, gender in the technocracy, the cultural roots of violence against women and paradigms of progress in corporate culture. Books in progress include* The Technocratic Body and the Organic Body: Hegemony and Heresy in Women's Birth Choices *and* The Power of Ritual. *Current research projects include the use of intuition by midwives and homebirthers; the paradigm shifts made by physicians from technocratic to holistic medicine; the aerospace industry's futures planning for the commercialization of outer space; and future directions in North American midwifery.*

This chapter is an abridged version of "The Rituals of Hospital Birth" in *Conformity and Conflict: Readings in Cultural Anthropology*, 8th edition, edited by James P. Spradley and David McCurdy. New York: HarperCollins, 1994.

Why is childbirth, a unique and individual experience for every woman, treated in such a standardized way in the United States? No matter how long or short, how easy or hard their labors, the vast majority of American women are hooked up to an electronic fetal monitor and an IV (intravenously administered fluids and/or medication), are encouraged to use pain-relieving drugs, receive an episiotomy (a surgical incision in the vagina to widen the birth outlet) at the moment of birth and are separated from their babies shortly after birth. Most of them also receive the synthetic hormone Pitocin to speed their labor, and give birth flat on their back. Nearly one quarter of them are delivered by cesarean section.

Most Americans view these procedures as medical necessities. But cross-cultural evidence does not confirm that they are. For example, the Mayan Indians of Highland Chiapas hold onto a rope while squatting for birth, a position that is far more physiologically efficacious than the flat-on-your-back-with-your-feet-in-stirrups (lithotomy) position. Mothers in many low-technology cultures give birth sitting, squatting, semi-reclining in their hammocks or on their hands and knees, and are nurtured through the pain of labor by experienced midwives and supportive female relatives. What then might explain the standardization and technological elaboration of the American birthing process?

One answer emerges from the field of symbolic anthropology, which encompasses the study of myth and ritual. As a long-time student of this field, I know that myths express the basic beliefs and values of a culture, and rituals enact and display those beliefs and values. In all societies, major life transitions such as birth, coming of age, marriage and death are times when cultures are particularly careful to display their core values and beliefs. Thus, these important transitions are so heavily ritualized that they are called *rites of passage*. Through these rites of passage, each society makes sure that the important life transitions of individuals can only occur in ways that actively perpetuate the core beliefs and values of their society. Could this explain the standardization of American birth? I believe the answer is yes.

I came to this conclusion as a result of a study I conducted of American birth between 1983 and 1991. I interviewed over 100 mothers, as well as many of the obstetricians, nurses, childbirth educators and midwives who attended them.[1] While poring over my interviews, I began to understand that the forces shaping American hospital birth are invisible to us because they stem from the conceptual foundations of our society. I realized that American society's deepest beliefs and values center around science, technology, patriarchy and the institutions that control and disseminate them, and that these core values are very clearly and effectively enacted and perpetuated through the high-tech obstetric procedures that have become standard in hospital birth. In other words, obstetric procedures are far more than medical routines: they are the rituals which initiate American mothers, fathers and babies into the core value system of the technocracy. The *technocracy* is what some anthropologists are calling American society in its current form.[2] A technocracy is a hierarchical, bureaucratic society driven by an ideology of technological progress. In the technocracy, we constantly seek to "improve upon" nature by altering and controlling it through technology.

Ritual works by sending messages in the form of symbols. Symbols are received by the right hemisphere of the brain, which means that instead of being analyzed intellectually, a symbol's message will be *felt* through the body and the emotions. Thus, even though recipients may not be consciously aware of the symbol's message, its ultimate effect can be extremely powerful. Routine obstetric procedures—the rituals of hospital birth—are highly symbolic. For example, to be seated in a wheelchair upon entering the hospital, as many laboring women are, is to receive through their bodies the symbolic message that they are disabled; to be put to bed is to receive the symbolic message that they are sick. Although no one pronounces, "You are disabled; you are sick," such graphic demonstrations of disability and illness can be far more powerful than words. One woman told me: "I can remember just almost being in tears by the way they would wheel you in. I would come into the hospital, on top of this, breathing, you know, all in control. And they slap you in a wheelchair! It made me suddenly feel like maybe I wasn't in control anymore."

The intravenous drips commonly attached to the hands or arms of birthing women make a powerful symbolic statement: they are umbilical cords to the hospital. The cord connecting her body to the fluid-filled bag places the woman in the same relation to the hospital as the baby in her womb is to her. By making her dependent on the institution for her life, the IV conveys to her one of the most profound messages of her initiation experience: in American society we are all dependent on institutions for our lives. The message is even more compelling in her case, for *she* is the real giver of life. Society and its institutions cannot exist unless women give birth, yet the birthing woman in the hospital is not shown that she gives life, but rather that the institution does.

Why would our society want to send such messages to women as they give birth? Because we have made a heavy investment in the *technocratic myth*. This myth insists that the more we control nature, the better it gets, and that ultimate control of nature is possible. Believing this myth, we have focused enormous energy on building machines that we can control in order to control nature, which we ultimately cannot control. But these powerful machines do generate at least the appearance of control. They help us to feel safe, and they extend our human powers enormously. So it is no wonder that we invest so much energy, attention and faith in them. Back at the beginnings of the industrial age, we were so impressed with mechanization that we even began to think of our own bodies as machines that could be taken apart and put back together to ensure proper functioning.

At that time, and for a long time after, it was commonly believed that women were inferior to men—closer to nature and feebler both in body and intellect. Consequently, the men who developed the idea of the body-as-machine also firmly established the male body as the prototype of this machine. Insofar as it deviated from the male standard, the female body was regarded as abnormal, inherently defective, and dangerously under the influence of nature. The metaphor of the body-as-machine and the related image of the female body as a defective machine eventually formed the philosophical foundations of modern obstetrics. Wide cultural acceptance of these metaphors accompanied the demise of the midwife and the rise of the male-attended, mechanically manipulated birth.

In keeping with the industrialization of American society, the rising science of obstetrics adopted the model of the assembly-line production of goods as its template for hospital birth. Accordingly, a woman's reproductive tract came to be treated like a birthing machine by skilled technicians working under semi-flexible timetables to meet production and quality control demands. As one fourth-year resident observed: "We shave 'em, we prep 'em, we hook 'em up to the IV and administer sedation. We deliver the baby, it goes to the nursery and the mother goes to her room. There's no room for niceties around here. We just move 'em right on through. It's hard not to see it like an assembly line."

The hospital itself is a highly sophisticated technocratic factory; the more technology the hospital has to offer, the better it is considered to be. Because it is an institution, the hospital constitutes a more significant social unit than an individual or a family. Therefore, it can require that the birth process conforms more to institutional than personal needs. As one resident explained, "There is a set, established routine for doing things, usually for the convenience of the doctors and the nurses, and the laboring woman is someone you work around, rather than with."

The most desirable end product of the birth process is the new social member, the baby; the new mother is a secondary by-product. One obstetrician commented, "It was what we were all trained to always go after—the perfect baby. That's what we were trained to produce. The quality of the mother's experience—we rarely thought about that."

Rituals are often repetitious, conveying the same message over and over again in different forms. The rituals of hospital birth remind women in several ways that their body-machines are potentially defective. These include periodic and sometimes continuous electronic monitoring, frequent examinations to make sure that the cervix is dilating on schedule, and, if it isn't, administration of Pitocin to speed up labor so that birth can take place within the required twenty four hours.[3] All three of these procedures convey the same messages over and over: *time is important, you must produce on time, and you cannot do that without technological assistance because your machine is defective.*

When humans are subjected to extremes of stress and pain, they may become unreasonable and out of touch with reality. Ritual assuages this condition by giving people something to hang on to that can keep them from "falling apart" or "losing it." When the airplane starts to falter, even passengers who don't go to church are likely to pray! To perform a ritual in the face of fear is to restore a sense of order and control to the world. Labor subjects most women to extremes of pain, which are often intensified by the alien and often unsupportive hospital environment. American women who believe in the technocratic myth will look to hospital rituals to relieve the distress resulting from their pain and fear. They utilize breathing rituals taught in hospital-sponsored childbirth education classes to restore a sense of order and control. They turn to drugs for pain relief, and to the reassuring presence of medical technology for relief from fear. When women who have placed their faith in the technocratic myth are denied its rituals, they often react with intensified fear and a feeling of being neglected. One woman recounted,

My husband and I got to the hospital, and we thought they would take care of everything. I kept sending my husband out to ask them to give me something for the pain, to check me, but they were short-staffed and they just ignored me until the shift changed in the morning.

I was terrified when my daughter was born. I just knew I was going to split open and bleed to death right there on the table, but she was coming so fast, they didn't have any time to do anything to me. . . . I like cesarean sections, because you don't have to be afraid.

When you come from within a belief system, its rituals will comfort and calm you. Accordingly, those women in my study who began labor in basic agreement with this technocratic (technological, interventionist) approach to birth expressed general satisfaction with their hospital births. They were the majority—seventy out of one hundred, or seventy percent. Their numbers are not surprising, as their profound distrust of nature and their faith in technology mirror the attitudes of our society as a whole.

In many cultures, to perform a series of rituals in precise order is to feel yourself locking onto a set of "cosmic gears" that will safely crank you through danger to safety. For example, obstetricians and many birthing women believe that correct performance of standardized procedures ought to result in a healthy baby. Such rituals generate in humans a sense of confidence that makes it easier to face the challenge and caprice of nature. However, once those "cosmic gears" have been set into motion, there is often no stopping them. A "cascade of intervention" occurs when one obstetric procedure alters the natural birthing process, causing complications, and so inexorably "necessitates" the next procedure and the next. Many of the women in my study experienced such a "cascade" when they received some form of pain relief, such as an epidural, which slowed their labor. Then Pitocin was administered through the IV to speed up the labor, but Pitocin very suddenly induced longer and stronger contractions. Unprepared for the additional pain, the woman asked for more pain relief, which ultimately necessitated more Pitocin. Pitocin-induced contractions, together with the fact that the mother must lie flat on her back because of the electronic monitor belts strapped around her stomach, can cause the supply of blood and oxygen to the fetus to drop, affecting the fetal heart rate. In response to the "distress" registered on the fetal monitor, an emergency cesarean is performed. Elise describes her experience of this "cascade of intervention":

> It's funny—it seems so normal to lie down in labor. Just to be in the hospital seems to mean to lie down. But as soon as I did I felt that I had lost something. I felt defeated. And it seems to me now that my lying down tacitly permitted the Demerol, or maybe entailed it. And the Demerol entailed the Pitocin, and the Pitocin entailed the cesarean. It was as if, in laying down my body as I was told to, I also laid down my autonomy and my right to self-direction.

The electronic fetal monitor is a machine that uses ultrasound to measure the rate of the baby's heartbeat through electrodes belted onto the mother's abdomen. This machine has become *the* symbol of high technology hospital birth. Observers and participants alike report that the monitor, once attached, becomes the focal point of the labor. Nurses, physicians, husbands and even the mother herself become visually and conceptually glued to the machine, which then shapes their perceptions and interpretations of the birth process. One woman described her experience this way: "As soon as I got hooked up to the monitor, all everyone did was stare at it. The nurses didn't even look at me anymore when they came into the room—they went straight to the monitor. I got the weirdest feeling that *it* was having the baby, not me." This statement illustrates the woman's internal acceptance of the technocratic myth that she is dependent on the hospital and its technology to give birth. Soon after the monitor was in place, she requested a cesarean section, declaring that there was "no more point in trying."

Internalizing this technocratic myth, women come to accept the notion that the female body is inherently defective. This notion then shapes their perceptions of the labor experience, as exemplified by one woman's story:

> It seemed as though my uterus had suddenly tired! When the nurses in attendance noted a contraction building on the recorder, they instructed me to begin pushing, not waiting for the *urge* to push, so that by the time the urge pervaded, I invariably had no strength remaining but was left gasping and dizzy. . . . I felt suddenly depressed by the fact that labor, which had progressed so uneventfully up to this point, had now become unproductive.

Note that she does not say "The nurses had me pushing too soon," but "My uterus had tired," and labor had "become unproductive." These responses reflect her internalization of the technocratic notion that when something goes wrong, it is her body's fault. Such an idea could only arise in a society that values machines more than bodies and institutional routines more than individual needs. Consider the visual and kinesthetic images that the laboring woman experiences—herself in bed, in a hospital gown, staring up at an IV pole, bag and cord, staring down at a steel bed and huge belts encircling her waist, and staring sideways at moving displays on a large machine. Her entire sensory field conveys one overwhelming message about our culture's deepest values and beliefs: technology is supreme, and you are utterly dependent upon it.

Once the woman's cervix reaches full dilation (ten centimeters), the nursing staff immediately begins to exhort her to push with each contraction, whether or not she actually feels the urge to push. When delivery is imminent, she must be transported, often with a great deal of drama and haste, down the hall to the delivery room. Lest the baby be born en route, the laboring woman is then exhorted, with equal vigor, *not* to push. Such commands constitute a complete denial of the natural rhythms of her body. They signal that her labor is a mechanical event and that she is subordinate to the institution's expectations and schedule.

Despite tremendous advances in equality for women, the United States is still a patriarchy. It is no cultural accident that ninety eight percent of American women give birth in hospitals, where only physicians, most of whom are male, have final authority over the performance of birth rituals—an authority that reinforces the cultural supervaluation of patriarchy for both mothers and their medical attendants. Nowhere is this reality more visible than in the lithotomy position. Despite years of effort on the part of childbirth activists, including many obstetricians, the majority of American women still give birth lying flat on their backs. This position is physiologically dysfunctional. It compresses major blood vessels, lowering the mother's circulation and thus the baby's oxygen supply. It increases the need for forceps because it narrows the pelvic outlet, making pushing more difficult, and ensures that the baby, who must follow the curve of the birth canal, quite literally will be born heading upward, against gravity. But it is very convenient for the physician, who has a clear view at a height that is comfortable for performing interventions. Thus it reinforces his status relative to the woman's—she is "down," and he is "up." If she were standing or sitting up to give birth, as many women do in other societies, he would be below her, bending to serve her—a radical departure from the cultural status quo.

The episiotomy performed by the obstetrician just before birth also powerfully enacts the status quo in American society. This procedure, performed on over ninety percent of first-time mothers as they give birth, expresses the value and importance of one of the technocracy's most fundamental markers—the straight line. Through episiotomies, physicians can deconstruct the vagina (stretchy, flexible, part-circular and part-formless, feminine, creative, sexual, nonlinear), then reconstruct it in accordance with our cultural belief and value system. Doctors are taught (incorrectly) that straight cuts heal faster than the small jagged tears that sometimes occur during birth, and that straight cuts will prevent such tears. But in fact, episiotomies often cause severe tearing that would not otherwise occur. Such teachings dramatize our Western belief in the superiority of culture over nature. Moreover, since surgery constitutes the ultimate form of manipulation of the human body-machine, it is the most highly valued form of medicine. Routinizing the episiotomy, and increasingly, the cesarean section, has served to raise the status of obstetrics as a profession, by ensuring that childbirth will be not a natural but a surgical procedure.

Nine percent of my interviewees entered the hospital determined to avoid technocratic rituals in order to have "completely natural childbirth," yet ended up with highly technocratic births. These nine women experienced extreme dissonance between their previously held self-images and those internalized in the hospital. Most of them suffered severe emotional wounding and short-term postpartum depression as a result. But fifteen percent did achieve their goal of natural childbirth, thereby avoiding being influenced by the technocratic myth. These women were personally empowered by their birth experiences. They tended to view technology as a resource that they could choose to use or ignore, and often consciously subverted their initiation process by replacing technocratic symbols with self-empowering alternatives. For example, they wore their own clothes and ate their own food, rejecting the hospital gown and the IV. They walked the halls instead of going to bed. They chose perineal massage instead of episiotomy, and gave birth like "primitives," sitting up, squatting, or on their hands and knees. One woman, confronted with the wheelchair, said "I don't need this," and used it for a luggage cart.

This rejection of customary ritual elements is an exceptionally powerful way to induce change, and indeed, many hospitals have responded.

During the 1970s and early 1980s, the dominance of the technocratic myth in the hospital was severely challenged by the natural
childbirth movement which these twenty-four women represent.
Birth activists succeeded in getting hospitals to allow fathers into
labor and delivery rooms, mothers to birth consciously (without
being put to sleep), and mothers and babies to room together after
birth. They fought for women to have the right to birth without
drugs or interventions, to walk around or even be in water during
labor (in some hospitals, Jacuzzis were installed). Prospects for reducing the influence of the technocratic myth by the 1990s seemed
bright.

Changing a society's belief and value system by changing the rituals that enact it is possible, but not easy. To counter attempts at
change, members of a society may intensify the rituals that support
the status quo. Thus a response to the threat posed by the natural
childbirth movement was to intensify the use of high technology in
hospital birth. During the 1980s, periodic electronic monitoring of
nearly all women became standard procedure, the epidural rate shot
up to eighty percent, and the cesarean rate rose to nearly twenty five
percent. Part of the impetus for this technocratic intensification is the
increase in malpractice suits against physicians. The threat of lawsuit
forces doctors to practice conservatively—that is, in strict accordance
with technocratic standards. As one of them explained:

> Certainly I've changed the way I practice since malpractice be-
> came an issue. I do more C-sections . . . and more and more
> tests to cover myself. More expensive stuff. We don't do risky
> things that women ask for—we're very conservative in our ap-
> proach to everything. . . . In 1970 before all this came up, my
> C-section rate was around four percent. It has gradually
> climbed every year since then. In 1985 it was sixteen percent,
> then in 1986 it was twenty three percent.

The money goes where the values lie. From this anthropological
perspective, the increase in malpractice suits emerges as society's effort to make sure that its representatives, the obstetricians, perpetuate our technocratic core value system by continuing to transmit that
system through birth rituals. Its perpetuation seems imperative, for

in our technology we see the promise of our eventual transcendence of bodily and earthly limitations—already we replace body parts with computerized devices, grow babies in test tubes, build space stations, and continue to pollute the environment in the expectation that someone will develop the technologies to clean it up!

We are all complicitors in our technocratic system, as we have so very much invested in it. Just as that system has given us increasing control over the natural environment, so it has also given doctors and women increasing control over biology and birth. Contemporary middle-class women *do* have much greater say over what will be done to them during birth than their mothers, most of whom gave birth during the 1950s and 1960s under general anesthesia. When what today's mothers demand is in accord with technocratic values, they have a much greater chance of getting it than their sisters have of achieving natural childbirth. Even as hospital birth still perpetuates patriarchy by treating women's bodies as defective machines, it now also reflects women's greater autonomy by allowing them to distance their minds from those defective body-machines.

Epidural anesthesia is administered in about eighty percent of American hospital births. So common is its use that many birth practitioners are calling the 1990s the age of the "epidural epidemic." As the epidural numbs the birthing woman, eliminating the pain of childbirth, it also graphically demonstrates to her the truth of the Western belief that mind and body are separate, that the biological realm can be completely cut off from the realm of the intellect and the emotions. The epidural is thus the perfect technocratic tool, serving the interests of the technocratic myth by enacting it, and of women who find meaning in that myth by enabling them to divorce themselves from their biology. Elaine said, "Ultimately the decision to have the epidural and the cesarean while I was in labor was mine. I told my doctor I'd had enough of this labor business and I'd like to . . . get it over with. So he whisked me off to the delivery room and we did it." For many women, the epidural provides a means by which they can actively witness birth while avoiding "dropping into biology." Explained Joanne, "I'm not real fond of things that remind me I'm a biological creature—I prefer to think and be an intellectual emotional person." Such women tended to define their bodies as tools, vehicles for their minds. They did not enjoy "giving in to biology" to be pregnant, and were happy to be liberated from biology during birth. And they welcomed advances in birth technologies as extensions of their own ability to control nature.

In dramatic contrast, six of my interviewees (six percent) insisted "I *am* my body," an chose to give birth at home under an alternative, holistic mythology which tells a very different story. It stresses the organicity and trustworthiness of the female body, the natural rhythmicity of labor, the integrity of the family and self-responsibility. The holistic story sees the safety of the baby and the emotional needs of the mother as one, and holds that the safest birth for the baby will be the one that provides the most nurturing environment for the mother.[4] Said Ryla, "I got criticized for choosing a home birth, for not considering the safety of the baby. But that's exactly what I was considering! How could it possibly serve my baby for me to give birth in a place that causes my whole body to tense up in anxiety as soon as I walk in the door?"

Although homebirthers constitute only one to two percent of the American birthing population, their conceptual importance is tremendous. Through the alternative rituals of giving birth at home, they enact—and thus guarantee the existence of—a story about pregnancy and birth based on the value of connection, just as the technocratic myth is based on the principle of separation. The technocratic and holistic myths represent opposite ends of a spectrum of beliefs about birth and about cultural life. Their differences are mirrored on a wider scale by the struggles between technomedicine and holistic healing, and between industrialists and environmentalists. These groups are engaged in a core value conflict over the future—a struggle clearly visible in the profound differences in the rituals they daily enact.

Obstetric procedures can be understood as rituals. These procedures are profoundly symbolic, communicating messages concerning our culture's deepest beliefs about the necessity for cultural control of natural processes. They provide an ordered structure to the chaotic flow of the natural birth process, appearing to contain and control it. And they strongly affect the birthing woman's perceptions of her experience. As one woman succinctly sums it up: "It's almost like programming you. You get to the hospital. They put you in this wheelchair. They whisk you off from your husband, and I mean just start in on you. Then they put you in another wheelchair, and send you home. And then they say, well, we need to give you something for the depression. [*Laughs*] Get away from me! That will help my depression!"

Through hospital ritual procedures, obstetrics deconstructs birth, then reconstructs it in ways that work to confirm the technocratic myth and to transmit the core values of American society to birthing women. From society's perspective, the birth process will not be successful unless the woman and child are properly socialized during the experience, transformed as much by the rituals as by the physiology of birth.

NOTES

1. The full results of this study appear in Robbie Davis-Floyd, *Birth as an American Rite of Passage* (Berkeley: University of California Press, 1992).

2. See Peter C. Reynolds, *Stealing Fire: The Mythology of the Technocracy* (Palo Alto, CA: Iconic Press, 1991) and Robbie Davis-Floyd, *Birth as an American Rite of Passage,* Chapter 2.

3. In Holland, by way of contrast, most births are attended by midwives who recognize that individual labors have individual rhythms. They can stop and start, can take a few hours or several days. If labor slows, the midwives encourage the woman to eat to keep up her strength, and then to sleep until contractions pick up again.

4. For summaries of studies that demonstrate the safety of planned, midwife-attended home birth relative to hospital birth, see Robbie Davis-Floyd, *Birth as an American Rite of Passage* (Berkeley: University of California Press, 1992), Chapter 4, and Henci Goer, *Obstetric Myths Versus Research Realities: A Guide to the Medical Literature* (Westport, CT: Bergin & Garvey, 1995).

Chapter 4

Preparing for Labor and Delivery
Andrea Frank Henkart

Prenatally it is important to select a birth plan that supports your belief system and to gain the support and cooperation of those assisting
you. The following guidelines suggest basic ways to take responsibility for your body, your birth and your baby, to ensure a healthy and
positive birth experience.

CREATE YOUR BIRTH TEAM

First, you must interview more than one care provider. Ask key
questions, and see what kind of response you get, and how your
questions influence their attitudes. Some care providers will welcome
your questions and encourage you to ask more. Ideally, a mutual respect will be formed, and the care provider you have hired to work
for you will assist you in achieving your goals. Others might be of-
fended or try to patronize you. Your current gynecologist may not be
the right obstetrician for you. I have known women who have
changed doctors in the last few weeks of pregnancy because the doctors were not living up to their promises.

Pregnant a second time, Linda asked her obstetrician what she
could do to avoid a second cesarean section. He patronizingly asked
why she would even consider "such nonsense." After much debate,
he finally agreed to a "trial of labor." Linda told him she didn't want
to be "tried" and decided to have her second child at home with a
midwife who was confident and supportive of Linda and her goals.

While in her seventh month of pregnancy, Adrienne told her obstetrician she was seeing a chiropractor who had suggested she take a

natural prenatal vitamin than the one he had given her. Her
flew into a rage, insisting, "I am responsible for you; I know
what is best for you. You can't see two doctors at the same time."
Not wanting to upset her doctor or make him angry, Adrienne re-
lented. After her baby was born, Adrienne told me that during labor,
her obstetrician kept insisting that "he knew best." During lengthy
prenatal discussions they agreed on many things. He told her she
could walk around during contractions, yet during labor when she
asked if she could get off the bed and walk around, he felt it would
be better if she remained still. Prenatally they had agreed that squatting was a great position to use during pushing. When she asked if
she could squat, her doctor replied, "I'd really prefer if you'd just lie
down on the bed. It's much easier for me to monitor you and your
baby." Prenatally, her doctor agreed not to perform an episiotomy,
yet while Adrienne was pushing, the doctor made a long cut along
her perineum instead of supporting it. When he was sewing her up,
he told her the episiotomy made it much easier for him to get the
baby out and was no big deal. "You'll heal right up; don't even
worry about it." This particular birth is not a rarity. I have seen this
kind of scenario happen time and time again.

The chief international medical organization, the World Health
Organization, supports the utilization of midwives as primary birth
attendants. Why don't we? Midwives have been the traditional birth
attendants since the beginning of time. Many of these strong, capable, knowledgeable, loving women bring years of tradition and "her-
story" into their profession. They see birth as a normal, natural
event. In fact, according to most midwives I have spoken with, many
use alternative techniques to ease and facilitate pregnancy and childbirth. Some of these alternatives include the use of nutritional counseling, herbs, homeopathic medicine, hypnosis, affirmations and
body positioning during labor. These techniques are often learned
through years of study and apprenticeship. Many of these safe and
proven alternative techniques are unknown to the medical profession! Jean, a childbirth educator who was studying in nursing school
to become a certified nurse midwife, told me, "Everything is techno-
logically and medically oriented. My curriculum *does not* include
natural birth."

A midwife from Holland wrote to me about home birth.

We have a special population of women; most of them want to
deliver at home. She feels safe at home, and we promote that.

But the first important thing is that we have a good relatio.
between gynaecologists, nurses and midwives. When you w
to create a change from hospital to home birth, first the trainir.
of the midwives must be changed. When it is normal for midwives and gynaecologists to deliver at home, and when there
are nurses who assist you at the delivery and continue their help
for one full week after the delivery, then there shall be more
home deliveries.

Stoppard (1993) says, "A planned home birth can be one of the
safest ways you can give birth." A recent British report has concluded that although ninety four percent of all births take place in
hospitals, they are no safer and may be less safe, than home births. In
Australia, a study of 3,400 home births found a lower perinatal mortality rate, and less need for cesareans, forceps delivery and suturing
for an episiotomy or a tear than in women delivering in hospitals.
The mothers were not all "low risk": the figures included fifteen
multiple births, breech deliveries, women who had previous cesareans and women with previous stillbirths. The group as a whole was
older than the national average. Less than ten percent had to transfer
to a hospital. Stoppard says that home birth in the United States is
more difficult. "Arranging a home birth isn't always easy or straightforward, but it's always exciting!"

If you decide to choose a midwife, interview more than one to find
the person who will offer you the kind of prenatal care you want and
support you in creating the safest, most gentle birth experience possible. Find out what her background is as a midwife and the kind of
setting in which she practices. Ask her what requirements you will
have to meet to be eligible for her practice, and let her know what
you expect in your birth. Because midwives provide services that depend on communication and preventive measures, you can lower
your chances of receiving an unnecessary cesarean by choosing a
qualified midwife as your birth attendant. Of all the births I have
witnessed, the most gentle, tender, loving births were in home situations with midwives in attendance.

Don't choose your doctor because he or she was nice even though
you had a cesarean, or just because you trust your sister's choice of
doctors, or your best friend recommended someone who she thinks
is great, or the doctor has known you all of your life. Trust your gut-
level instincts. Use your better judgment. Challenge your care
providers with questions about their personal belief system on child-

birth. Question their time limits for labor and second stage pushing. Find out what they honestly think about the importance of bonding with your newborn. Your doctor or midwife will be with you during a most intimate, exhilarating and emotional time. Choose someone you really believe in and who really believes in *you*.

THE CHILDBIRTH ASSISTANT

After you have hired your primary care provider, the next step would be to hire a professional childbirth assistant. Scientific researchers studying birthing women have begun to document benefits of continuous social support in labor. Klaus, McGrath, Robertson and Hinkley (1991) have reported that this continuous support significantly reduces medical costs by reducing the incidence of medical interventions, such as epidural anesthesia, cesarean section, Pitocin augmentation and forceps delivery. They say, "The challenge is to turn to obstetric technology only when necessary, relying instead on the practice of continuous labor support to help the birth process follow its natural, normal course." From my experience as a certified childbirth assistant for more than ten years, I have seen how having this kind of support can bring a proper perspective back to one of life's most incredible miracles: Birth! Childbirth assistants, like doctors and midwives, vary greatly in their personalities, techniques and fees. Paulina Perez and Cheryl Snedeker, authors of *Special Women: The Role of the Professional Labor Assistant* (1990), provide the reader with heartwarming stories of how women assist women in childbirth. They offer advice for supporting the father or partner, and precise information regarding how to deal with hospital, home or birth-center birth.

With the support of a professional childbirth assistant, your birth experience can be greatly heightened. The knowledge and personalized care your childbirth assistant provides throughout your baby's birth increase your self-confidence and feeling of security. Women with special needs or health risks and single mothers can all benefit from the support, guidance and expertise a birth assistant can offer.

Physicians and midwives have found that their job is often made easier by the presence of a childbirth assistant. When your medical team needs to focus on the more technical aspects of birth, the childbirth assistant is there to provide continuity of emotional support. The birth assistant can also be an invaluable help to your labor partner (also known as "the coach") by providing information and encouragement. Allowing your labor partner to relax and feel comfortable with the natural process of birth relieves him of all anxiety and possible pressure to perform. Some partners struggle to learn all the material from childbirth classes. Some never seem to have enough time to read all the books and hand-outs. Your partner may have an agenda of his own about birth, which he is uncomfortable telling you about because he does not want to worry you or scare you; after all, you are the one who is going to "do it."

Childbirth classes in America are very fixed on preparing our male partners to be coaches. In sports, coaches call the shots and solve the problems. With a proper job description in hand, these men are ready to lead us through the battle with flying colors. When those first strong contractions come upon you as a surprise, and you look at him with a sense of fear or concern or possibly even pain in your eyes, he may forget about what you wanted. Now he wants to save you. I have seen a man withdraw completely from a laboring woman because he was confused. In contrast, some men may use their machismo force to coerce their partner to have pain medication or a cesarean because it will get rid of the pain. In this way they can be in control, fix the problem and make the pain go away. With only the doctor to talk with in quiet whispers outside the delivery room, these two "partners-in-crime" make arrangements for you, prepare time schedules for your baby, figure out ways to "protect" you, and plot to make it all easier for you.

It is important for you to feel supported in labor. You must have the knowledge and inner strength to advocate for yourself. You must have a team of people surrounding you who don't give up at the slightest discouraging sigh from you. A slight dip in fetal heart tones may not be the end of the world. You need someone who can gently remind you and your partner that you are powerful, aware, and able to speak up for yourself. Communication skills are of the utmost importance between you and your birth team.

Some women and men may balk at the idea of having an "intruder" in the room during this most intimate time. Men often say, "I'll be there for her; she doesn't need anyone else." When a woman is in the throes of labor, writhing or screaming through the ritual of childbirth, she needs someone who can and will remind her to stay in her body, to stay with each contraction. The nurse on duty may be fully capable of offering labor support, but what happens if her shift ends in the middle of your contraction? When a woman in labor says, "I can't do this anymore," I say, "You *are* doing it. You are doing it right now." I also remind her that the contraction she thought would rip her apart has just ended. "*That* contraction will never come back again."

While a husband or partner may be very loving and supportive during labor, I have seen women turn away and not listen or believe her partner when he offers suggestions or words of advice. The relationship is often too intimate in many ways for her to really hear him, or she may doubt his knowledge of the birth process. Sometimes the messages must come from outside her own system to be heard fully. A childbirth assistant who has established a relationship with the woman prenatally and who stays with her from the onset of labor to the birth of the baby can be the one who helps the mother with the birth process while freeing the partner to offer more caring support.

Pregnant women should see their childbirth assistant at least two to four times prenatally. Each visit lasts approximately one to two hours. This differs greatly from the fifteen minute prenatal visits scheduled by the obstetrician. During these non-medical prenatal visits, the childbirth assistant will help you to create or fine tune your birth plan. As you become very clear about your own philosophy of childbirth and your upcoming labor and delivery, the childbirth assistant will begin to understand your beliefs and have a clear sense of your uniqueness and life-style. In addition, the time you spend together will allow her to know your emotional, physical and spiritual needs. Fostering confidence, trust, respect, education and non-medical comfort measures, she can help you adapt to your particular birth experience.

There are many different types of childbirth assistants. Claudia Lowe, the director of the National Association of Childbirth Assistants (NACA, 1992) defines a *professional childbirth assistant* as someone who is specifically "trained to provide skilled non-medical support for pregnancy, labor, birth, recovery, and postpartum." According to Lowe, a qualified childbirth assistant "can help a woman and her family create a positive birth and parenting experience."

Typically, a *labor coach* will meet the laboring woman at the hospital. The support she offers is provided during the actual labor and birth; prenatal visits are usually not included. A *doula*, the Greek word for servant, has taken on new meaning. In the beautiful book *Mothering the Mother* (1993), Klaus, Kennell and Klaus say a doula "has now come to mean a woman experienced in childbirth who provides continuous physical, emotional, and informational support to the mother before, during, and just after childbirth." A qualified childbirth assistant who assists the mother when labor begins and assists after the baby is born can help to increase maternal-infant interaction and gives the mother time to relax.

The training level of the different types of birth assistants varies greatly and will determine the level of care you receive. The professional should remain current in her field. Some certifying bodies require recertification every few years. The more comprehensive the service she provides, the more comprehensive her training should be. Some of the national and international organizations that train and certify childbirth educators and assistants are listed in the Sources of Further Information at the end of this book.

CREATE YOUR BIRTH PLAN

By creating a birth plan your team of "helpers" (your doctor or midwife, your birth assistant and the others in attendance—who are *all* your "hired help") will have a clear understanding of your needs. This birth plan should be designed according to your particular goals and desires. Do not be afraid to be assertive. Of course, all the requests should be reasonable for normal, healthy birth, which also includes VBACs. I encourage women to include a section on cesareans should one become necessary. Go over your birth plan with your childbirth assistant. She should be skilled enough to help you fine tune it, and carry it out while avoiding any adversarial situations with your care providers.

If your birth ends in a cesarean, you can still hold your baby immediately after the birth. You can have rooming-in in recovery. And while you are there, you can breast-feed and your baby can be held by your partner. Just let the hospital staff know what you want by stating it in your birth plan. You deserve to claim your own power in birth and do it your way. A birth plan is not a setup for failure, nor is it cast in stone. It is a way for you to empower yourself by taking responsibility for creating the birth you want. In addition, it is a tool for communication between you and your birth team and can be revised by you at any time as your pregnancy and delivery unfold.

I recommend that women look at the extensive birth plan in *Silent Knife: Cesarean Prevention & Vaginal Birth After Cesarean* (Cohen & Estner, 1983, p. 303) and rewrite it according to how they envision their birth to be. *Silent Knife* is an excellent resource for providing well documented information on everything from ultrasound to amniocentesis to management of the newborn. A pamphlet entitled *Planning Your Baby's Birth*, by Penny Simkin and Carla Reinke (1980), offers suggestions and methods for creating a birth plan, in addition to making choices in childbirth, becoming informed, and preparing for the unexpected. I have included a modified birth plan in the Appendices to get you started.

In preparing for a non-interventive birth experience, you must consider the baby's immediate experience as well. Do you want your newborn baby to be shipped down to the nursery? Do you want your baby to have a shot of vitamin K? Do you want your baby's heel pricked and blood drawn for various routine tests? What about erythromycin in the baby's eyes and the issue of circumcision? These all need to be addressed in your birth plan and given consideration before you give birth, so that your baby will not be subjected to any unnecessary medical procedures you may not want. Before our daughter was born, my husband and I researched all these topics very thoroughly before making any decision. Fortunately for us, we both agreed not to have any interventions if we could avoid them. Five and one-half years later when our son was born, we researched the issues again for new ideas, data, and statistics. Our research caused us to become even stronger advocates for non-intervention. *Mothering Magazine*, a quarterly publication, is rich with information on the latest health issues, in addition to child rearing, toilet training, immunization, positive discipline, and the art of parenting. Find out what will automatically be done to your baby after birth; do some research on the various interventions used. Most hospitals do not inform you of your rights as a pregnant patient. It is your newborn's right to be protected by you.

After your birth plan is written, discuss each line with your care provider. Have your care provider initial the points with which he or she agrees. By having care providers acknowledge each point line by line you are assured they will be true to their word, and not just provide lip service. The points that they cannot legally or medically endorse can be discussed so each of you knows where the other one stands and has an understanding of the other's belief system. Find out how your care provider manages postdate pregnancy, fetal distress and other possible concerns. How will your care provider support your perineum during second-stage pushing? Does your care provider feel comfortable with a breech birth? Prior to labor, find out which colleague (if any) may substitute for your care provider.

Discuss your birth plan with any potential substitutes. Communication skills are vital to consumer advocacy.

Be sure that a copy of your birth plan is included in your medical file at all times, and submit copies to your hospital or birth facility, doctor or midwife. Mailing your birth plan to the labor and delivery unit of your local hospital makes it very easy for that very important document to get lost somewhere in the hospital paperwork. I strongly recommend you hand deliver it to the head nurse during one of your hospital tours or during pre-registration, to make sure it goes directly into your file. It is important to note that in a hospital setting, nurses must follow hospital regulations. If you are planning a hospital birth, having your birth plan in your file in advance will allow the hospital staff to work toward the objectives you and your primary care provider have previously agreed upon. Be sure your childbirth assistant has a copy before labor begins. By having a pre-assigned list of what is important to you, your birth assistant can support you to the fullest of her ability.

EDUCATE YOURSELF

Read, read and read some more! I have included many excellent books in the Bibliography. Don't limit yourself to those listed, but do beware of books which can lure you into believing that a medically oriented birth is completely painless, guiltless and easier. *The Complete Book of Pregnancy and Childbirth* by Sheila Kitzinger (1993), *The Birth Book* by Sears and Sears (1994) and *Conception, Pregnancy and Birth* by Dr. Miriam Stoppard (1993) are all beautifully written books with wonderful photographs that cover topics such as exercise, nutrition, the pros and cons of medical interventions and just about everything you need to know about pregnancy, labor and delivery. *Open Season: A Survival Guide for Natural Childbirth & VBAC in the 90s* by Nancy Wainer Cohen (1991) is a comprehensive, occasionally irreverent, informative and powerful book that shines a light on unnecessary interventions and gives women confidence in their ability to birth naturally. *Heart & Hands: A Midwife's Guide to Pregnancy & Birth* by Elizabeth Davis (1987) and *Special Delivery* by Rahima Baldwin (1986) are two older books that I still recommend because they are easy to read, highly informative and they promote gentle childbirth.

It is vitally important to attend consumer-oriented childbirth classes. It is a well-known fact that when the classes are not doctor or hospital influenced, you will receive broader, more open insights to childbirth. Go to support groups and workshops on birth-related issues, especially if you believe the topic is something that you are sure "won't happen to me." Don't depend on your care provider, your childbirth assistant or your partner. Discover ways to feel confident within yourself. Depend on *you* and your baby.

TRUST YOURSELF

Typically, in America when a woman becomes pregnant she doesn't even realize it. She goes to her gynecologist for a test to confirm her suspicion. Once she is pronounced pregnant, the next words out of her mouth are typically "Now what do I do?" Following her doctor's advice, the woman usually does everything she has been told to do without asking "Why?" Pregnancy, labor, delivery and raising a family are not subjects taught in school. In fact, many women with vast educations, multiple degrees, and access to incredible knowledge do not even know how to tell if they are pregnant or how to diaper a baby once the little bundle arrives!

I urge you to take responsibility for yourself. I encourage you to learn about your baby and your changing body and acknowledge the ever-changing feelings that keep coming up. *Do not under any circumstances give your power away to anyone.* By this I mean, do not blindly follow the instructions of your obstetrician because you "trust him completely." Remember to ask questions, and trust yourself. A doctor who warns you that you might need a cesarean section, or that your baby is too big, or that you are too big needs to be questioned. Find out exactly what your doctor means by these potentially threatening diagnoses. Be responsible; surrender to your body and the baby taking it over from inside. *Trust in your Self and your body's ability to give birth naturally.* Giving birth is a beautiful, miraculous passage into motherhood and should *not* automatically be treated as a medical event.

Lisa, a psychologist pregnant with her first child at age 39, is planning a home birth. Lisa has been counseling families for many years, has worked extensively on her own personal growth and has a very loving, supportive relationship with her husband. She is well read and feels very prepared to offer her baby a gentle, non-traumatic birth experience. Lisa thought she had it all together, yet was disturbed by a lot of morning sickness and a feeling of general malaise. She contacted me "just to talk."

In our session together, Lisa told me that she believes in a strictly holistic approach to childbirth. She has "the best chiropractor, acupuncturist, homeopath and herbologist in California." She sees them all on a regular basis and feels like she is in control of her own body. With all of this positive assistance, Lisa feels confused. She wonders why she still vomits in the mornings, has dry heaves in the afternoon, and feels lousy the rest of the day. I reminded Lisa that she has a human being growing inside her body. That would cause anyone's body to feel different! I also reminded her that as her hormones were rapidly changing, her baby was feeding off her from the inside out. If she could just surrender to the miraculous process of growing a human being inside herself, she just might let go and be able to relax into her body instead of fighting the feelings that come with pregnancy.

When I asked her to tell me about something she did for herself that felt good, she told me that she is still working full time but took a day off to go to the beach. Feeling ecstatic, Lisa walked along the beach with the swell of her belly gently protruding from her bathing suit.

As we continued to talk, I discovered that Lisa finds her job to be very stressful. She really wanted to take more time for herself and wanted to take her maternity leave early. She felt guilty about the thought of leaving her clients and staying home while her husband was out working all day. Through continued exploration, Lisa came to the conclusion that some of her malaise was due to pent up anger about giving but not being able to receive. What she really wanted to do was sleep late every morning, take a daily walk on the beach, and prepare for labor day. Lisa was actually longing to be with her baby, but was not allowing herself to take the time to *feel* the process of pregnancy and motherhood.

Becoming a mother begins in pregnancy. You must take care of the baby growing inside of you. Go for long walks, cuddle in bed holding your baby-belly, and allow yourself to feel the presence of the child within while you ease into the role of mother. A woman often needs this time to get used to the idea that she is transforming into a mother. If you already have children, this pregnant time allows you to prepare for the increasing fullness of your mind, body, spirit and home. Prepare yourself well as you await for the emergence of this new being. When labor day arrives, it will be easier for you to fully embrace and surrender to the process of giving birth.

When labor does begin, stay home as long as is safely possible. Stay active, walk, take a hot shower, or take a nap if you can. Do whatever you can to remain comfortable. Having your birth assistant there to assist you will greatly relieve any anxiety you may experience. Having reviewed labor support techniques prenatally, fine-tuned your communication skills and gained a clear understanding of the process of labor, you will know exactly when it is time to go to the hospital or call your midwife. If you are going to have a hospital birth, I cannot overemphasize the importance of staying home in early labor.

Just about every time I hear another cesarean story, or a "horrible" birth experience, it is because the birthing couple did not have a professional childbirth assistant to guide them, and because they checked into the hospital too soon. Getting there early in labor may cause you to become more anxious, and it just gives the hospital more time to "set you up," which may make you more susceptible to an unnecessary cesarean section. By this I mean, hooking you up to various monitors, excessive vaginal exams, and Pitocin augmentation if labor appears "slow" by their schedule, making you feel like a patient instead of a woman in the midst of a miracle.

I have found that fetal distress is often related to maternal distress. When mothers in labor become nervous, frightened or confused, their fear level rises which causes an increase in adrenaline, and consequently the stress level of the baby may rise as well. The adrenaline goes to the baby as it crosses the placenta and can induce fetal distress.

This was true for Caren while she was in labor with her first child. She had been at the hospital for hours. Caren's doctor gave her an ultimatum upon her arrival, "Either you have your baby within twelve hours, or I'll need to consider doing a cesarean." He explained that he felt it was important she deliver quickly so the baby would not be compromised. (According to Caren's medical records, when this diagnosis was given in early labor, there was no apparent danger to the baby.) Caren was very conscious of the clock looming overhead as it ticked the minutes away. Approximately nine hours into her labor, the doctor came into the room. After checking her cervical dilation, he told her that he was going off duty and that his partner would take over. Caren became confused and concerned, as she didn't really know her doctor's partner very well. The second doctor decided to use a few medical interventions to "ease her own mind." Caren tried to argue, but flat on her back in labor was not the best time to start a debate. As Caren became fearful, her blood pressure went up. She started to cry, so the nurse administered oxygen. As all this was happening, there was an immediate drop in fetal heart tones. Caren's birth assistant leaned toward her. She put a protective, loving arm around the laboring woman and whispered gently into her ear. She reminded Caren to use her own inner power to remain centered. She encouraged Caren to go within herself, to talk to her unborn child and let her body do what it needed to do despite the confusion and anger. Amid all the chaos of nurses scurrying around like busy ants, and the doctor throwing orders about, there came an immediate recovery of heart tones for the baby, and lowering of blood pressure for the mother. The head nurse turned to the birth assistant and, shocked, asked, "Whatever did you say to her?" The International Cesarean Awareness Network literature says, "Try a 'tincture of patience' and remember a long, slow labor may be normal for you."

When preparing for labor and delivery, the process does not end with creating a good birth team. The process continues on. . . . Before and during labor it is important to be forewarned about routine hospital procedures that have thrown many women off their guard. Entering the hospital for a "natural" birth, Janet was shocked to find that her initial requirement of fifteen minutes on the fetal monitor turned into twelve hours of hook-up with the inability to get up and move with her contractions. Pitocin augmentation upset Glynnis and caused her to give up on the gentle, slow labor she had planned for herself. Her doctor said she was taking too long and the baby may be fatiguing. When she said she wasn't really that tired and also knew her baby was strong, her doctor replied, "We can't take any chances." Was it the baby at risk or the doctor's malpractice insurance? When discussing the use of routine episiotomy in vaginal delivery, Dr. Allen (not his real name), told me, "Off the record? I cut 'em all. Makes it easier for me, the baby and the mom. I can sew her up in no time and she's fine for the wear and tear." It is because of the outrageous overuse of monitors, machines, slicing, augmenting and convincing that I believe women should be informed about some very common hospital procedures used during labor and delivery.

UNNECESSARY EPISIOTOMIES

To prevent tearing or unnecessary cutting of the perineum (the area between your vagina and anus) during second stage labor, it is important to strengthen your pubococcygeus muscle prenatally. The pelvic floor muscles support your uterus, bowel and bladder. During pregnancy, the pelvic floor muscles tend to relax due to an increase in progesterone. By doing the Kegel exercise at least twenty five times a day, you can strengthen and tighten the muscles, providing you with a supple perineum. Lift your vaginal canal upward toward your torso; pulling and tensing the muscles as if you were consciously stopping the flow of urine. Hold the upward movement as long as you can and release very slowly. You can do this exercise anytime and anywhere.

A strong perineum may prevent the often unnecessary and much overused episiotomy. An episiotomy is a cut made into a woman's perineum to enlarge her vaginal opening. In her book *Conception, Pregnancy & Birth* (1993), Dr. Miriam Stoppard says, "This is an overdone, often unnecessary surgical procedure." She also says, "Episiotomy is the most commonly performed operation in the West" and "[c]ommon child-bearing myths have it that there are no nerve endings in the perineum and that a woman is bearing so much pain anyway as the head is born that she will not feel the pain of episiotomy. This is utter nonsense and nothing less than brutal." It is interesting to note that the Scandinavian countries have a five percent episiotomy rate while the United States episiotomy rate is ninety-six percent! Some doctors still tell women that they will "stitch them up so their vaginas will be tight as virgins." Debra worked long and hard for her VBAC. She sadly stated, "But I still didn't escape the surgeon's knife. He cut me all the way down to my rectum. I should start a new group called the Episiotomy Prevention Movement!" With proper perineal massage and support, attention to body positioning while pushing, and pushing to the rhythm of body and baby, I have found that most women *do not* need to have their bodies cut to bring their children into this world. In an interview with Beatrijs Smulders, a practicing midwife in Holland, Ali Crolius (1992) found that Dutch midwives regard episiotomy as ritual mutilation. Smulders says, "It's the final word by doctors that you really can't do this without our help."

Upright positioning during pushing can aid the force of gravity and may allow your perineum to stretch. Massaging the perineum with pure vitamin E, or olive oil, and applying warm compresses to the perineum while pushing may prevent tearing or the need for cutting. Ask how your care provider will support your perineum so you can efficiently push your baby out.

Some women feel that an episiotomy is "no big deal." A woman in labor may say, "If that's all they want to do to me, then let them do it. It's better than a cesarean." It is this kind of attitude that supports the routine use of this procedure. Nancy Wainer Cohen (1991, p. 106) refers to episiotomy as "crotch-slicing." If an episiotomy is not medically necessary, don't "let them do it" to you. How do you know if your perineum needs slicing at the last minute? A vaginal opening does not need enlarging. It will open and stretch all by itself, and with proper support, you won't necessarily even tear. There are no studies to prove that a cut is better or safer than a tear. However, your care provider may give you reason to believe that episiotomy is the best alternative. Cohen goes on to say, "Episiotomy has nothing to do with the adequacy of the perineum—only with that of the care provider. Providing care does not include slicing our genitals."

I have been told by many women that their tears have healed easily, with no complications. Kitzinger (1990) has shown that complications such as excessive bleeding and infection are quite common when the perineum has been sliced. You have a right to keep your body intact.

AVOID UNNECESSARY PITOCIN AUGMENTATION

Women constantly talk about their babies being late, as if the babies did not understand the importance of deadlines! According to Kitzinger (1991), due dates given at the beginning of pregnancy are just a statistical mean. She says, "Studies show that only five percent of babies arrive on that day."

If your baby is past due, your care provider may have numerous tricks for bringing on labor before your baby and body start the process automatically. Angelica, a nurse midwife from San Francisco, California told me,

Each doctor has his or her own order for bringing on labor or just checking to see if everything is okay. They usually start with a fetal monitor in the hospital to check the heartbeat of the baby or they send the mom home to check how many times her baby kicks in a certain given time period. That one is so dumb because sometimes the baby is sleeping! If they still want more information on the status of the baby, they might do a sonogram. Sometimes the doctor will break the amniotic sac to see if that brings on labor. Or they just hook the mother up to a Pitocin drip to see if contractions start. I have rarely seen a mom go home from the hospital once this procedure starts. They always promise her she can go home after they check things out, but she never leaves. The Pitocin usually makes the contractions hard, long and strong. This increases muscle tension and her maternal stress level, which both work against her. She needs to be able to relax so her uterus will work unimpeded.

Oxytocin is a natural hormone released from the brain to stimulate labor. Pitocin is the synthetic hormone used to induce or stimulate labor. It is administered through an intravenous drip so you must remain in bed on your back. I have seen women receive Pitocin augmentation to "get those contractions going," and in many cases it does help them to birth quicker. But the routine use of this "drug" is not always necessary. In the case of a medical emergency, machines and medication can save lives. A study by Ettner (1979) consistently concluded that these interventions can also stop or slow down the process of normal labor, in addition to causing complications to the baby.

From my experience with women in labor, I have found these alternatives to Pitocin to be most beneficial:

- Look into your own psyche and emotions to see where you may be holding back.
- Honor and respect your baby's time schedule by allowing your baby to "fully cook."
- Walk prenatally to tone your entire body in preparation for labor.
- In labor, do nipple stimulation to release the body's natural oxytocin.
- Homeopathic remedies can often prevent lengthy and painful labor.
- Warm water in the form of a bath, shower, or warm compresses can be miraculous in reducing the pain of contractions, and assist a laboring woman to relax, refreshen and open up.

Empowering a laboring mother to trust in her ability to relax and believe in her body's own time schedule may be the only medicine needed. If all these techniques still don't work and the laboring mom does need Pitocin, she can still maintain her dignity and her desire to continue with the remainder of the birth in the most natural way possible. Don't "throw in the towel" and give up on all previous plans. A positive attitude and trust in your body's ability to *open* is crucial.

FETAL MONITORS

According to Hausknecht and Heilman (1991), there are two kinds of monitors used in labor. The internal fetal monitor (IFM) is an electrode which attaches into the baby's scalp. The external fetal monitor (EFM) consists of two straps which are placed around the mother's pregnant belly. Both types of monitors provide a continuous recording of the fetal heart rate, and an assessment can be made as to whether the unborn baby is in distress. Gabay and Wolfe (1994) have shown that the rise in the rate of cesarean sections corresponds directly to the routine use of the fetal monitor.

In his book *Birth after Cesarean* (1990), Dr. Bruce Flamm states, "Fetal monitors only test the baby's heart rate" (p. 76). He goes on to imply that the event of true fetal distress is rare. He then provides the reader with an amusing story of an "adult monitor," which is hooked up to an adult patient, and measures how fast his heart is beating. The "adult" is left in a darkened room and is never seen or examined by the doctor; he is merely "monitored" from outside the room. This "adult monitor" cannot measure pulse, blood pressure, or temperature or analyze urine. In this situation the doctor cannot tell much about the adult's state of health; in fact, the doctor cannot even tell whether the adult is sleeping! Dr. Flamm correlates the absurdity of this "adult monitor" with the current use of fetal monitors. He further states, "Fetal monitors have no doubt saved the lives of many babies, but fetal monitoring is a very inexact science" (p. 77).

Although constant monitoring is useful in high risk pregnancies, most mothers and babies do not require it. Fetal monitors have become a high-tech replacement for the fetoscope, which resembles a stethoscope. Stoppard (1993) says that fetal monitors "increase the amount of electronic equipment in the delivery room, making the atmosphere very clinical, and the staff may concentrate more on the machine than on you. Because attendants are aware of any tiny changes that may occur, they are more likely to intervene rather than letting labor take its natural course over time."

Mary was having a vaginal birth after cesarean in the hospital with a very progressive obstetrician as her attendant. When Mary told him she did not want any interventions during this birth, he agreed by initialing *everything* she had requested on her birth plan. As Mary entered the birthing room the nurse on duty told her to undress and lie down so she could attach the external fetal monitor (EFM) to her protruding belly for the obligatory fifteen minutes of monitoring. When Mary told the nurse that she would remain in her street clothes for awhile and had no desire to lie down, the nurse started talking about hospital policies and protocols. As Mary's birth assistant, I gently reminded the nurse to check the birth plan that was on file. Much to the surprise of the nurse, the doctor had left orders to use a fetoscope instead of the EFM to check the baby's heart tones. The nurse laughed and said, "I haven't used one of those things in years, this will be interesting!" The labor proceeded with love, support, patience and time. The energy in the room remained calm and unhurried. No one ever shouted, *"push!"* Mary released her daughter out of her vagina at her own pace as she squatted on the bed, while her obstetrician supported her perineum. Mary went home that evening. The next day I returned to the hospital to talk to the nurse. She said,

> I thought about that birth all night. I've been a labor and delivery nurse for twenty five years and have never really seen a birth like that one. At first I was so mad that *I* had to get uncomfortable to listen to the baby's heartbeat. I prefer the fetal monitor. It's so easy to just watch, then I don't have to pay so much attention to the mother. But this birth was so different. Everyone was so calm and quiet, it was like an angel being born. And we didn't use anything! That's the part I can't believe. No monitors, no drugs, no forceps, no episiotomy, no nothing! I just can't believe it. And for a VBAC yet! I guess I've become really jaded over the years. I'm so used to all those machines. Listening to that heartbeat with my own ear during her labor made me feel humble. I can't really explain how I felt. I haven't cried at a birth in a long time, you know I see so many. But this one was special. This one felt like we all just helped that mom do it herself, and I guess that's just how it should be.

If you are in labor and medical procedures do become necessary, know your options. If you make conscious, educated decisions based on every possible bit of information you have obtained, then the choice remains yours. Technology does not have to spoil your personal experience in giving birth. Labor can be an overwhelming and dramatic experience. The powerful tightening produced by contractions may be painful, but this pain has a greater purpose. Prepare yourself emotionally, mentally and physically so you can approach labor and delivery with complete confidence.

Simple Tools for an Easier Labor

- *Prenatal yoga* is a great way to tone, firm up and stay in conscious contact with your unborn child. I recommend reading Jeannine Parvati Baker's book *Prenatal Yoga & Natural Birth* (1986), and *Natural Pregnancy* (1990) by Janet Balaskas. They both give a complete description of exercises and meditations for pregnancy and childbirth. You can use many of the postures to help you through labor. Prenatal yoga will calm you and increase your awareness of your baby, bringing you a sense of peace.

- *Relaxation* through visualization, prenatal massage, emotional support, comfortable positioning, gentle stroking or soothing, and any other stress-reducing technique can help a woman in labor let go and open up. Pregnant women often complain of being unable to relax. Massage on a regular basis throughout your pregnancy can help you to release tension, allows you time to tune in to your baby, and gives you that time to yourself that you deserve. The feeling of relief and relaxation can be your prenatal gift to yourself. A professional massage therapist, your partner or a close friend can rub your back, your feet, your arms and your neck. During labor, massage can help to reduce pain and stress. It can also help you to stay centered in your body and focused on your baby.

- *Get plenty of rest.* At least two weeks before your estimated due date, start paying close attention to your body's need for sleep. Nap when necessary, and get all the sleep you can at night. You would not run a marathon without the preparation your body needs. Exhaustion in labor can often lead to a cesarean section. Going into labor well rested helps tremendously. When a woman becomes exhausted in labor, she may need assistance from various drugs or machines. As a result of the overuse of these various drugs and machines, a woman may give up trusting herself and her baby. Her new-found lack of trust coupled with an increase in fear may provoke her into an operation to help her give birth. Listen to your body and take time to sleep.

- *Eat* little snacks during labor to keep your energy up so you don't succumb to exhaustion. A midwife told me that by increasing your complex carbohydrate load to sixty-five percent of the calories you take in one week before your due date, you will create a greater storage of glycogen in your muscles, so you can last that much longer when you do finally go into labor. In the early phases of labor before your cervix is half dilated, eat easily digested foods like soup, vegetable and fruit purees or tea with honey. Avoid milk and high fiber foods. In strong labor your stomach shuts down, but can still absorb glucose. Keep giving yourself natural boosts as needed.

- *Stay well hydrated.* One rule of thumb is to take a sip of water or juice after each contraction, or suck on juice-flavored ice chips. This reduces your need for intravenous fluids, which, once all the tubes are hooked up to you, will prevent you from moving around as freely as you might want.

Chapter 5

Accept the Process: A Commentary on Childbirth Education

Gina Maria Alibrandi

Gina Maria Alibrandi has a B.A. in Art History and a B.S. in Nursing. Specializing in Maternal-Child Nursing, including obstetric and gynecologic care, she has worked in the birthing field since 1978. She is a licensed Registered Nurse, a Public Health Nurse, a Certified Childbirth Educator, a retired La Leche League Leader, and the mother of three children, all born at home. Having worked with medical doctors, certified nurse midwives, and direct entry midwives, she is a parent and baby advocate functioning within the medical system.

Through her childbirth preparation classes, Ms. Alibrandi has prepared thousands of couples for birth and the transition to early family life. She has provided direct guidance and support to hundreds of women during the birth process, both within and outside of the hospital setting. In addition, she has written numerous articles and given presentations on the subjects of pregnancy, birth and lactation.

She believes deeply in the value of childbirth education, having witnessed first hand the results which stem from either the presence or lack of preparation for this major turning point in life. She currently works as an R.N. at the only free-standing birth center in Northern California and is in high demand for the childbirth preparation classes which she teaches within her community. Ms. Alibrandi received a research grant to examine the relationship between prenatal breastfeeding education and maternal satisfaction with breastfeeding. A book on fetal development for the lay person is forthcoming.

Childbirth education is a process that begins with one's own birth and continues throughout life. How a growing girl, a woman-to-be, is told of her own birth, *if* she is told, will influence her attitude about this miraculous process for her entire life. This education continues throughout life. The way in which menstruation is explained to an adolescent has the potential to fill her with pride in the marvel that is her body, or with shame. Childbirth education is a cultural process, a process which until recently was portrayed in a fearful way by most Western societies.

Most women of childbearing age have grown up in an era when the media portrayed birth as a frightening, painful, life-threatening process. With such fear-filled images connected with childbirth during a woman's developing years, it is no wonder that many modern women have a difficult time letting go, to allow unhampered labor to bring their children into this world. Fortunately, some of these media images are less frightening today for young women-to-be (the pregnant mothers of our future).

If childbirth truly required technological intervention, there would not be a birth explosion in developing countries. Worldwide most births take place outside hospital settings, at home, under trees, in caves or in grass huts. In Africa, !Kung women leave their group and go off by themselves to have their babies in the bush. To require the assistance of another while giving birth would cause a !Kung woman to feel ashamed. They are able to birth alone because the childbearing process has been designed by nature, over thousands of years, to be largely successful when it is left alone and allowed to pass in its own time. These women giving birth in their natural setting trust in the perfection of their bodily processes. They not only accept the rigors of labor but embrace the effort of childbirth for the wonderful outcome that comes forth.

The human body is a truly marvelous piece of machinery. The living body grows, heals itself and reproduces. One does not need to think about the minute by minute biological processes which take place. One simply accepts that the lungs expand, the heart beats and oxygen is then carried to every cell. In the same way, with the innate intelligence present in the body of a laboring woman, a child is brought forth into the world. The miracle of life remains an undiscovered secret. Babies are conceived and born daily all over the world to people who simply accept the process without analysis or fear.

The natural order of life is to reproduce and create future generations. Without reproduction, civilization and humanity would cease. In this context it makes no sense for reproduction to be an arduous process requiring technical expertise to succeed. If human birth truly required medical expertise and a sterile environment, then our beloved species would have died out hundreds of thousands of years ago. We must remember that a woman's body is beautifully designed to nourish, protect and bring forth the next generation. When an infant is ready for life outside the womb, a signal originates from the fetus that helps to initiate the powerful uterine contractions of labor. The intense work of labor builds until it crescendos with the welcoming of a baby into this world. As a newborn emerges from the body of its mother, a casual observer cannot help but be awestruck at this miracle of life, and the marvelous work of the woman's body through this process.

In the past, having a baby was accepted as a natural event, a part of nature, like the flow of the tides and the phases of the moon. Explanation of childbirth was handed down from mother to daughter. Birth was a part of everyone's developmental experience as people had large families and young women gave birth in their home or the home of another family member. Girls coming of age helped with the birth of their loved ones, and were present when their mothers, sisters, aunts, cousins and neighbors had babies. While recognized as an arduous and sacred process, childbirth was also commonplace. A woman pregnant for the first time already had secondhand experience of the ebb and flow of labor. She knew that she should expect arduous work and that labor would probably hurt. She also knew that she could count on the support of the women in her community to provide her with massage, hot and cold compresses, herbal teas and other comfort measures when her time came to embark on the journey of motherhood.

The birth of a baby was a joyous event, accompanied by great celebration and tremendous pride felt by the entire extended family and community. Giving birth, like the tilling of the fields, was accepted as hard work and well worth the effort. After the birth, the new mother was still cared for by her loved ones as she and her new child got to know one another. Childbirth education took place in the context of day-to-day living. A class covering how to breathe in order to get a baby out of its mother and what to do with the baby once it was out would have seemed an insane idea in such a climate of community knowledge, support and love.

Rather than a continuous cultural education for birth, many newly pregnant couples today seem to think of childbirth education as a series of "Lamaze" classes. In these classes they often expect to learn a variety of complicated breathing techniques which they hope will enable childbirth to proceed without pain. One woman said that during her first pregnancy, she thought she *had* to take Lamaze classes or else it would be physically impossible for her to give birth. It is a sad statement of our cultural attitudes about childbirth that many women believe that they are physically unable to give birth unless they attend a formal childbirth preparation class. The uterus already knows how to birth a baby. The mother takes classes only to "learn" to accept the process and trust her body.

Childbirth education as a set of specialized classes is an aberration in history. Societies which live closer to nature and the biological processes would probably consider the idea of taking classes to learn to give birth to be as silly as taking classes to learn to eat and to defecate. Many modern couples expecting a child for the first time have never even witnessed the birth of domesticated pets, let alone a human birth. Because they lack any exposure to normal childbirth, it is no wonder that people are anxious about what lies ahead for them in the birthing process. It is natural to be frightened by the unknown.

Sadly, the feminine knowledge of how to give birth has been lost in recent generations. This practical and gentle information is no longer passed from mother to daughter in most instances. Formalized childbirth classes for expectant mothers and their partners represent an attempt to revive the cultural knowledge necessary for women to give birth. The value of childbirth education classes lies in the potential to enable a pregnant woman to understand intellectually a powerful natural process in which she soon will be engaged. Thus, prepared childbirth classes are an attempt to create a substitute for the lifelong lack of exposure to the birth process.

Through understanding childbirth, a woman can more readily yield to that process rather than resist the efforts made by her body. The use of relaxation techniques, usually one facet of childbirth classes, allows a woman in labor to respond without resistance to the strong sensation accompanying a uterine contraction. This allows her uterus to work unhindered by bodily tension. Often, people raised in our fast-paced society have not learned to be quiet and peaceful within themselves. For many people, it is necessary to practice relaxation and breathing techniques in order to achieve a state of generalized relaxation.

Childbirth education classes vary greatly in their quality and orientation. Some hospital-sponsored classes consist of a tour of the maternity ward, along with an explanation of routine medical interventions. The opposite extreme consists of classes that are midwifery mini-courses, complete with details about fetal cellular biology and physical assessment. Still other classes resemble stress management classes with little explanation of the workings of the body and little, if any, information on consumer advocacy. Ultimately childbirth education should be a process of acceptance. Learning to accept the fear of childbirth, physical pain and the unknown of future parenting can be achieved by some without the format of a structured class. Others respond best to the support provided by a formal class structure.

Overall, childbirth education classes seem to be valuable for the majority of expectant mothers in contemporary society. Not only do the mothers and their partners become familiar with the unknown, but parents-to-be also meet others who are experiencing similar feelings associated with this process; this takes away the sense of isolation felt by many expectant mothers. A woman generally brings someone to class who will serve as her "labor coach," often the father of the child. In class a woman prepares for her pending labor while the labor companion learns techniques to provide her with support. Many women have said that they would not have been able to get through labor without the continual support and encouragement provided by their companion(s).

Do not hesitate to shop for a birth class that will provide a broad base of information and birthing "tools." Many people put more thought into the purchase of an automobile than they do into their decisions related to childbearing. An auto can always be sold. A woman's memories of birth will last a lifetime. It is important to be thoughtful and create the safe and special birth experience that is desired, regardless of the chosen setting. Selecting a compatible childbirth educator is part of this process. There are many certifying groups for childbirth educators, along with various techniques provided by instructors even within the same certifying body. Many childbirth educators continue to follow one method of childbirth preparation, particularly Lamaze or Bradley. In my experience, the best classes offer a continually evolving eclectic mix of effective methods, along with guiding a woman in finding what works best for her. A smattering of information on consumer advocacy within the often intimidating medical field is also useful.

The various relaxation and breathing methods taught are generally based on successful labor experiences of large numbers of women.[1] Different instructors teach different breathing techniques. Decide what works for you. The type of birth class is not as important as the orientation of the individual instructor. Be sure you interview the instructor. Does the instructor encourage a woman to find her own way to relax and achieve comfort? Does the class discuss medical interventions and their life saving abilities as well as their possible side effects if unnecessarily applied? Does the instructor make an effort to teach the class participants how to communicate and work with, rather than against, the health care providers involved? Many hospital-based classes are oriented to prepare patients for the hospital's routine, rather than to help gear the hospital to meet the needs of individual laboring women. For this reason many women find that private classes, taught away from the hospital, are usually more consumer oriented, and the material is often presented with a greater degree of objectivity.

By allowing herself to accept and embrace the hard work and pain of labor, a woman also allows herself to experience intense joy, excitement, frustration and the satisfying exhaustion that accompanies physical exertion. Before a woman can accept what will happen to her in labor and birth, she usually needs to first understand the labor and birth process. A thorough class will explain the anatomy and physiology of the birth process using diagrams and models with plenty of time for questions. There may need to be a considerable amount of cultural unlearning to be done by the class as well, depending on past exposures and experiences. Negative statements heard while growing up such as, "I almost died from the pain when you were born" can be replaced with positive imagery such as, "Giving birth is the most powerful and uplifting work a woman can do," or "Sure, it hurts, but look at the lifetime of laughter and joy that comes forth from that effort."

Negative conditioning about childbirth received throughout a lifetime can be altered with positive childbirth education during pregnancy. Classes, books, and speaking with women who are positive about their birth experiences all help to reinforce a healthy, balanced view of birth. More important than any amount of knowledge about the mechanics and politics of childbirth, the ability to relax and stay centered within one's inner core is the ultimate tool to manage the rigors of giving birth. This ability to relax deeply and find an inner core of peace amid physical upheaval is the most important tool in facilitating labor.

Through conscious relaxation, a woman allows her uterus to work, unimpeded by self imposed stress and tension. Relaxation, acceptance and trust in the natural intelligence of the human body, with a bit of patience thrown in for good measure, are the most important tools to be gained through childbirth education, whatever form that education may take. Giving birth becomes much easier by accepting the powerful ebb and flow of labor. As a side benefit, this same relaxation and trust can also prove to be useful for helping one to cope with other processes in life.

As you learn to welcome each labor contraction with love, rejoice in the knowledge that its power brings your child closer to your loving embrace. Trust your body; accept and embrace the process.

NOTE

1. Breathing techniques are useful as means to help achieve relaxation of the voluntary muscles while fully oxygenating mother and baby. Breathing techniques do not, on their own, guarantee a swift and painless passage of the newborn through the birth canal.

Chapter 6

Visualization Techniques for Relaxation
Andrea Frank Henkart

In our hurried-up time of stress, work, family and home, Super
Woman finds herself so stressed she does not even have time to focus
on her pregnancy. In addition to her job, her family and her changing body, she now believes she has to buy everything sold in the local
baby store. "I have to finish the baby's room soon," she admonishes
herself. What Super Mother-To-Be doesn't realize is that her newborn only needs to be held, nursed and kept warm.

In times of stress, women can benefit from practicing relaxation
techniques at least once a day. For some women, the time right before falling asleep is the only time they allow themselves to relax.
However, any time is certainly better than no time at all. Relaxation
increases your coping skills, and can increase your comfort while
you are in labor. As your body relaxes, your pain tolerance increases. Relaxation techniques allow your abdominal muscles to
relax, which allows your uterus to contract more efficiently, and
you may feel more in control when you do not have to fight each
contraction.

Positioning your body is very important in maximizing your ability to relax. Find the most comfortable position, and change to another one whenever necessary. You can lie on your left side, recline
in a chair or in a warm bath with your knees bent, or sit on the
floor and lean back against a wall or your partner. However, do
not lie flat on your back, because your uterus will press on major
blood vessels which can reduce blood flow to the placenta. Use as
many pillows as you need to cushion and support your head, arms,
chest, abdomen and legs. During labor, you can relax by squatting

or holding on to your partner and bearing your weight down in the assisted squat position.

There are many types of relaxation techniques. The tensing and releasing of your muscles helps to consciously relax every part of your body. Prenatal massage allows gentle pressure to sweep away tension from your body. Yoga stretches your muscles and allows your energy to run freely. Meditation relaxes your mind as you consciously release negative thoughts. Imagery or visualization techniques can bring about pleasant, comforting sensations to your mind and body. What's more, many women have successfully turned their babies to a more favorable position using visualization techniques.

To master the art of visualization, you just have to be able to lie down and relax! You may want to record this visualization on an audio cassette and play it back to yourself. Or you can have someone read it to you very slowly and softly. You can even make up your own visualization.

Find a comfortable, quiet place where you won't be disturbed. Turn your telephone off, lower the sound on your answering machine, turn the lights down low. Loosen your clothing so you are very, very comfortable. Close your eyes and focus on your breathing.

Feel your body resting on the surface where you are lying. Feel the weight of your entire body. Notice your breath. Don't change your breathing in any way; just notice that as you inhale your stomach rises gently. As you exhale, your stomach relaxes and falls. Watch the natural rhythm of your breath. Like a newborn baby's, your breath flows easily and effortlessly. Remember, when you are in labor, you will breathe in deeply through your nose as your belly rises, and as your breath releases through your mouth, your belly will relax and sink in. This style of diaphragmatic breathing allows your diaphragm to expand as you inhale and balloons your stomach out so that your lungs can fully open, bringing clean, fresh air to your little baby nestled deep within your womb. As you exhale, your lungs contract, causing your diaphragm to push down as your belly sinks in like a deflating balloon, allowing all the stale air to be released from the depths of your body. Continue this process of slow, deep breathing.

Now imagine that a big ball of white light is gently hovering over your body. See that big ball of sunlight as it begins to illuminate your body. Feel the warmth of the sunlight as it penetrates through you into the very core of your being, illuminating the life within as you continue to gently breathe.

Allow the warm, comforting rays of warmth and light into your feet. Feel the weight of your feet on the ground. See your feet in your mind's eye illuminated with white light; feel the warmth of the light penetrating into each toe, tingling the soles of your feet. Repeat silently and slowly to yourself, "My feet are relaxed, my feet are relaxed, my feet are completely, completely relaxed."

Take a deep, cleansing breath and visualize your calves, your knees, and your thighs. See both of your legs illuminated with the warm light of the sun as it hovers gently over your body. Bring that warm light down, down, into your legs, filling them with a sensation of peace and comfort as you release, release, completely release your legs. Take another deep breath and relax.

Gently move your awareness now to your hips, buttocks, pelvis and vaginal area. See your entire pelvic area illuminated with the glowing, white light. Feel this warm-colored light illumine your pelvic floor. This area which has grown and softened during your pregnancy has been carrying and rocking your baby for many months now. Like a baby nestled safely in a papoose, so your baby is being cradled. Silently in your mind's eye, command your pelvis to relax, pelvis relax, pelvis completely, completely relax.

Visualize your back in your mind's eye now. Your lower back, your upper back, all along your spine. Allow the healing white light into your back as you feel the warm fingers of the powerful light rays begin to tickle upward on your spine. Knowing your back is inherently strong and is the backbone of your very being, allow your upper and lower back to let go just a little more. Feel each intricate muscle let go just a little more, as you feel your body sink farther and farther down into the ground. Command your back to let go as you release, release, completely, completely release your back.

Focus now on your belly. Deep within lies a little, tiny baby, your baby. Your baby is nestled safely inside you and continues to breathe even as your own breath has slowed down consid-

erably now. Your baby is growing right this very minute. The pattern for your child's body has already been decided. Your baby's hair color has already been decided. The intricate fingerprints of your tiny baby are deeply ingrained in the DNA of the little being growing within you right now. Illuminate your belly in your mind's eye now so that the warm, penetrating rays of the white light hovering over your body dance right into the space where your baby is growing. Feel the warmth spread over your ever-growing belly. As if you were in labor, surrender to your breath and allow your baby-belly to relax, belly relax, baby and belly completely, completely relax.

Slowly move the light into your shoulders. Allow the energy to flow right down your arms into your hands. See the white light flowing gently down, down your arms right into the very tips of your fingers. Move the energy through your hands into your fingers, and right out your fingertips. Relaxing your shoulders, arms, hands and fingers, repeat to yourself, "Relax, relax. Shoulders, arms and hands completely, completely relax." Take another deep, soothing breath and gently release it.

Continue working up your body until you see your neck and head illuminated with the glowing, white light. In your mind's eye, see all the intricate muscles in your neck swell with warm, healing energy. Move that energy into your head, onto your scalp and down every strand of hair on your head. Your head and neck are now completely illuminated with the warm, white light. With your eyes gently closed, your jaw loose, and the tip of your tongue resting lightly on the roof of your mouth, let go and allow your entire neck, head, scalp and face to completely, completely relax.

Breathe gently as you slowly become aware of your entire body resting lightly amid the cushiony pillows nestled around your body. Notice how slow your breath is now, almost as if it weren't even there. Feel the weightlessness of your body, like a cloud floating through the air. In your mind's eye, let your body float up like a cloud, as you soar above the trees, above the ocean, through the clear, blue sky. Notice how relaxed your whole body feels as you glide through the air. Your whole body is completely, completely relaxed.

Allow yourself five to ten minutes to relax. Let your thoughts wander without giving any attention to any particular one. Let each thought flow into the next. Give your mind

*and body the opportunity to release any stress. Breathe gently
and relax.*

*Ever-so-gently begin to bring your awareness back into
your body. Slowly begin to focus on the little tiny baby growing deep within your womb. Protected, cuddled and safe, I
want you to visualize the position of your baby. See in your
mind's eye just where the little head is situated within your
womb. Gently notice where the tiny buttocks and feet of your
sweet baby are. In your mind's eye, remember where you last
felt the kick of your baby's feet. Now, visualize the position
you want your baby to be in. See the little head down toward
your cervix, pressing right down onto your cervix. See your
baby's little head buried deep within your pelvis. Imagine what
it would be like if your baby followed each instruction easily
and effortlessly. Allow your baby to follow your guidance. Let
your baby begin to turn now, to turn so that the little head is
resting down in your pelvis. Prepare the position of your
baby's head to facilitate an easy exit. Tuck your baby's chin
right down onto its chest. Let your baby move easily and effortlessly within the walls of your womb. See your precious little one nestled safely within your womb, head down, feet up
toward your ribs. Remind your baby to tuck her little chin
right down onto her chest. This will put her head in an easy
exit position. Continue to see your baby in this way. Talk to
your baby, reassure your little one that she is safe, that her
birth will be gentle, joyous, and that you will be right there to
love and protect her. As you maintain these thoughts, let your
body relax even deeper, and breathe deeply. As you let yourself
just be, you can feel how you and your baby are one.*

*Very gently now, inhale deeply—expand your diaphragm,
filling it with air. Slowly exhale, contracting your lungs. Now
begin to move your fingers. Stretch them out wide; wiggle
them. Wiggle your toes; gently rotate your ankles. Very slowly
move your arms way over your head and stretch them. At the
same time, stretch your legs way down. Open your mouth very
wide, feeling all of your facial muscles come alive again. When
you are ready, open your eyes.*

Be sure you sit up very slowly. Wait a minute or two before you
go about your day. If you practice your visualizations before bed-
time, don't worry if you fall asleep. Once you have completed an

entire visualization process, it is often helpful to write down any thoughts or feelings that may have come up. These thoughts and feelings can be part of a journal, where you document the beginning of your baby's life. Some women give the journal to their children when they have grown into adults; others keep it as a personal account of this precious, emotional, special, often stormy time of personal growth.

Chapter 7

Body Wisdom: The Forgotten Information in Childbirth

Donna Germano

Donna Germano, M.A., MFCC, is a Licensed Psychotherapist and Specialist in Post-Traumatic Stress Syndrome and women's issues. She is one of the original founders of Hospice in America. In 1977, Ms. Germano co-founded a home-care hospice in the greater Los Angeles area to care for the dying and their families. She was a founding member of the first statewide Hospice Board in California, and a member of the Bio-Ethical Counsel for Christians and Jews concerned with human values in relationship to hospice care. During that time, she led support groups for those with life threatening illnesses and specialized in grief and bereavement counseling. For the past 12 years she has worked with men's and women's traumas from combat and with their families burdened with the secondary effects of war. In 1988, Ms. Germano went to the former Soviet Union to offer information about post-traumatic stress to Soviet psychologists and veterans of the Afghan War. She held the first informal women's group in Kazakstan for the effects of war on women and children. She is completing a forthcoming book, Tears of Men: The Gifts of Nam, *describing the legacy and transformation of men's war trauma and the hidden experience men have of body.*

Currently Ms. Germano is in private practice in the San Francisco Bay area and works with a wide range of people with trauma from events such as combat, accidents, catastrophic illness, surgeries and hysterectomies. The elements of trauma presented to her throughout her career have forcibly drawn her attention to the reality that the body has a life of its own, with its own primal intelligences and meanings that are perfectly oriented to survival and well being. She has learned to work with the body's own ageless resources to transform physical and emotional distress. She says, "Body has taught me what mind was too busy to hear."

The act of giving birth is one of the most elemental and primary activities in a woman's life. It certainly is the most essential activity to human life and is, fortunately, the furthest from being controlled by our conscious mind. For this reason, we have to re-learn what we have forgotten, how to relate to the life of our bodies. This life is instinctual and, because it is so basic, it has everything to do with gut reactions and deep emotions. The body has its own purposes and its own goals that are distinctly different from the way we think things should be. Like it or not, our bodies set the rules for our experiences. Definitely, the body has its own wisdom, yet we are usually unaware of this level of "intelligent" life within us.

Body life has been ignored and body wisdom is lost in this modern age that overly emphasizes the intellect, reason and abstraction and forgets or dismisses as not valuable the non-rational nature to which we are born. For this reason, when women give birth today they far too often have bad experiences and suffer long term effects that undermine their self-image, their self-confidence and, ultimately, their well-being. We are unaware that what happens to our bodies during childbirth will subtly influence other aspects of our lives afterward because the experiences our bodies go through are remembered not by our minds but by body memory. Many common experiences during childbirth today are actually interferences from the mechanical world, for example, the use of fetal heart monitors and of drugs to induce labor, which carelessly (though well intentioned) disrupt what our bodies have been instinctually doing forever. This interference is not given much thought or is dismissed as being non-consequential, because everyone else seems to think this way, but it doesn't change the alienating effects that the co-opting procedures have on our bodies. Even births by cesarean operation are treated lightly. But, in fact, everything done does matter; the life of the body is our real life, the only life we have.

Some awareness of your body's own life does come back to you when you begin changing throughout pregnancy and when labor begins. Then you find yourself immersed in the forces of the body, which have their own kind of intelligence and which—know it or not—are powerfully connected to the elemental force of life that has been evolving on this planet over many millennia. We do not usually think this deeply about having a baby, even though throughout the world pregnant women joke about their bodies no longer being theirs. It is only when we begin thinking about having natural childbirth or anesthetized births, what hospital to use, or whether to deliver at home that some awareness of life's forces comes to us. Knowing about this life of our body is important and valuable to help us during labor and afterward, because we can work with this life as it comes to us rather than being swamped by it. And it does come powerfully through physical sensations, such as pain and pressure, emotions such as rage or joy, and a host of feelings, images, and thoughts that accompany the physical experiences of labor.

"IT" IS THE PROBLEM

Among the chief reasons we have lost this knowledge of body wisdom is the negative attitudes and beliefs that our culture has about matter and about the life of the body. We have objectified ourselves, and our bodies have become *things*. This shows up most clearly when we try to talk about our bodies; we refer to our own body as "it," and become self-conscious and awkward when we try to find words to indicate that our bodies are indeed ourselves. Religion, science and family mores have taught us that we are separate from our bodies, that we are more than our bodies or not our bodies at all, and that our bodies are not really us but are something that we are supposed to discipline, train, use well or discard in favor of a higher state of being.

It is not possible to talk about the historical reasons for this strange distance from ourselves that we have invented without going far beyond the purposes of this writing. But it is important to know that this lost connection to our body's own wisdom greatly affects women throughout their lives and shows up particularly when women give birth, and when medicine, men, and machines take over and co-opt what has been nature's process for eons of time. Whether women choose to go with the ways of giving birth that medical and insurance industries consider right and correct, or whether they choose natural home births, or any variation of these scenarios, it is in our best interest as women to stay connected to our body's wisdom.

It is particularly damaging, and even dangerous, however, to be cut off from the world of our body's wisdom during pregnancy and labor. Labor pains can make us feel crazy and mad, sad or helpless, and we may want to give in to anyone else who would tell us what is best for us even though he or she is not having these birth experiences. Lying down during labor, for example, is something your body would want to do only when it needs temporary rest, and most of the time it is the body's urge to move, push, hit, squat and discharge as much energy as it can while laboring to deliver the baby. The desire to lie down in labor is not in your body's best interest for the many reasons cited in numerous books on childbirth.

There is much we can learn about ourselves when we begin to listen to the signals and cues our body gives us about what it needs and what makes it work best, when we are going through the stages of labor. By paying attention to ourselves as body and not just personality, we can make a big difference in how we experience childbirth, and how we feel about our lives and our bodies after birth.

There is a lot to be aware of when your body begins to change over to creating another human life. At the onset of this process, many women get a sense that there is something different in their bodies even before they miss a period, but they cannot quite describe the difference. As pregnancy progresses, the changes in the body are pronounced and unmistakable to see on the outside, but the intelligence of the body also changes. The body adapts to the inherent creation pattern it follows and goes into an ageless rhythm of withdrawal from life on the outside, into the deep processes of life that are going on inside. The first clue of this rhythm is the tiredness, or spaciness, or reveries, or restlessness that come over a woman from time to time in the early stages of pregnancy. All of the changes in body and mood during pregnancy come from the influence of ancient patterns of life being stirred in a woman's body.

Most women acknowledge this without having words for it and take it in stride. However, that can mean that women also will not respond to their bodies and will ignore the gathering forces of life that will prepare her for the time of labor and delivery. All the cues for how to relate to our bodies during labor are beginning during this time, showing up as all those tiny and mysterious mood shifts, energy fluctuations, and aches, and the myriad sensations that come from all parts of our body. Without abandoning the necessary chores or jobs women have to do, time and space must be made for women to begin listening to these clues, for they are the advance heralds about how labor and delivery will take place. The language of the body is clear long before labor begins; staying strongly connected to it during labor is essential to a good birth, whether you are delivering naturally or not.

Amazingly, when a woman goes into labor, the life of the body is not taken into account by those attending the birth: what is accounted for are the external authorities, medical technologies, protocols, and correctness of what birthing *should* be like to be right. But curiously, the body, the woman's body, is no longer the major focus of birthing. It has subtly shifted to being a secondary thing, something that must be acted upon and intervened with. Great importance is put instead on the medical knowledge, outside interventions, and medical authorities who believe they know how things should be according to technology. Organic process—nature—is considered less trustworthy or safe than "rational methods" such as the use of anesthesia, fetal heart monitors, and cesarean section, which are available to take over for the body when birth does not go the way we (or they) think it should.

THE BODY

The body not only knows about itself and what it needs to function, but reacts to experiences that happen to us and stores them as emotions, feelings, reflexes and body memory. Our basic instincts keep us alive, functioning and moving lifeward until we eventually die. This is the normal cycle of life and our bodies know how to live it. The most obvious ways we see it are, for example, common everyday events. Your stomach will let you know if you have eaten something that does not agree with you. Should you insist on repeating the experience, your stomach may rise up in rebellion. In fact, the entire body will come to the stomach's aid, and many other systems will give off messages that what is happening should stop. Minimally, you might get gastritis, halitosis, diarrhea and a headache, or at worst, land in an emergency room desperately ill. Our bodies always give us cues about what is needed, what is not, what is helpful to its goals and what opposes those goals. We just don't know how to listen.

When a woman goes through labor, memories and emotions arise and are released as our bodies begin to contract, push, release and gather momentum for the next contraction. Physical sensations of pain and pressure are often accompanied by an emotional experience that sometimes takes the form of old emotions such as fear, sorrow, grief, anger and helplessness. These emotions will not matter if a woman feels connected to her own body, if she trusts her body, and if she lets her body take over. During the most intense part of labor, a woman's emotions blend with the physical, and body and imagination are one. She is both completely vulnerable and extremely powerful all at the same time, in which the entire range of human potential—from the purely instinctual, to the emotional, to the rational—comes the closest it can to a single focused unity. In giving birth, a woman actively experiences the most primary force of life and, in so doing, keeps the feeling of life alive.

That is one reason it is best if women remain awake, aware and actively participating in the birth process, rather than being zonked out with anesthesia and drugs. If we take the medical and medicated route, the release of body memory and emotions happens nonetheless. At a deep basal level the body has its own instincts for survival and taking care of itself, and when labor begins, all the experiences of life, harmful or pleasurable, are deeply recalled at a low level of awareness. Whatever experiences might have been harmful will arise in the body memory and inject themselves into the process of labor, making some of us wild with fear and eager to shut down to what is going on in our bodies.

On the other hand, pleasurable memories stored in the body can make birthing become the orgasmic experience many women report that it has been for them. This body memory can arise anywhere during the labor process, at the onset, while riding out strong intense contractions and even during the last phase when delivery is beginning. The experience of our lives begins to tie into the deeper primal pulse of life as birthing comes to its climax.

At this point, the body will "talk." It may make no logical sense, but it is there. The birth attendants may notice many signs that the woman in labor is going through something powerful that has to do with her and the life forces. She moves, grunts, laughs, wails, pants, and lets her animal nature move out of her—if she is lucky enough to have social and mental support for her movements and sounds. At the onset of labor, the ancient instincts of childbirth begin to take over. At this time, the very best move a woman can make is to respond to her body's need to move in certain ways. That might not be completely possible if she is hooked up to machines (alarming in itself), but whatever movement can possibly be made should be allowed. Sound is energy, too, and is an important part of the way the body moves energy. Our bodies make their intentions known at times like these, and being alert to what they might be is helpful. Our bodies can be a safeguard against the infringements of technology in the birthing process.

REMEMBERING

Bodies carry the memory of life on earth, of all forms of life, of the mineral and elemental world, and the reality of what matters. All of this might be of no interest to us until the time comes when we suddenly have to be back in our bodies in a big way, as in childbirth. This is true not only of birth, but in situations that cause us to be traumatized such as a bad car accident, the loss of a limb, or being in battle.

Maybe we could let ourselves trust what goes on with our bodies more fully if we realized that we have within us an automatic and unconscious knowledge to stay alive. All of our body's sensations are information about what is going on with it, what its needs are, and how to interact with the world around us.

We are three brained ones, and two of our brains, the most ancient ones, are the results of the countless eons of evolutionary survival on this planet. They have within them the memory patterns of every stage life has passed through throughout the ages and are involved in everything to do with staying alive, surviving, being well, protecting ourselves, keeping the species going, bonding, nurturing and giving pleasure. It is from these brains that we get our emotions and feelings, and our drive to live.

We are not aware of this part of our brain structure because popular psychology emphasizes only the functions of the two hemispheres of our newest brain and says nothing about the life of the body. This bias is reflected clearly in the things we do when it comes to giving birth, and the things we don't even think to do, such as taking cues from the body about itself and the processes that it puts us into during labor.

There are times when a laboring woman thinks that she might lose it, that the whole birth process is beyond her, and she hates what she is going through. My sister-in-law's reaction to her laboring of many hours was an angry frustration: she was "not going to do this anymore" and she was "going home" from the hospital. We had to prevent her from leaving and remind her that she was having a baby!

Reasonable and humorous at the same time, she reacted to body wisdom that told her to move and to get a different attitude about her process. She was going to please herself—her body—even in those circumstances, and moving to make herself more comfortable was the key. The moving she was doing was actually all she needed to do even as the baby was crowning. It was the movement, a shift in mood and energy, and a ferocious determination to *do* something that resulted in a sudden, quick delivery.

Far too often, when we come to a point where we totally lose it in labor in a hospital birth or at home, we don't remember that the body is wise and is constantly giving us information that we can act upon to help us. We become afraid and want to run. That is exactly when we must stay in our bodies, face any panic and learn from it. We tend to forget that the body knows what the process is, that the body always compensates and recompensates on the verge of life; otherwise what women go through in childbirth would be intolerable. It is only when we do not remember or forget to face our bodies that we tend to run. This is true even if we are hooked up to a machine or need emergency attention.

We may need help remembering how to stay connected to our own body wisdom. Too often those who love us cannot help us because they also have forgotten, and because it is not easy to see the one they love in any kind of pain. It is possible to forget why you are where you are. Remember: you are going to have a baby.

All we need to do is remember the body's wisdom from time to time. Just remember.

Chapter 8

When Push Comes to Shove:
What to Do if You Have a Cesarean
Andrea Frank Henkart

When a woman does have a cesarean, she often is confused, scared, feeling like a failure and in great pain. Basic information for recovery is generally not given before surgery. Typically, the cesarean information and complications class offered during many childbirth courses is the very one that a pregnant woman will miss.

Immediate care begins in recovery. Waking up from a general anesthetic can be somewhat alarming and severe pain is usually felt right away. According to Hausknecht and Heilman (1991), the nurse most likely administers a painkiller, usually from the Demerol or morphine family. These drugs can produce a sleepy, hallucinogenic or "spaced out" feeling. As the medication wears off, sometimes women feel nauseous. The fear of vomiting after major abdominal surgery is common, not to mention feelings of anxiety, disturbance of internal organs and hormonal changes.

Epidural and spinal anesthesias tend to wear off much more gradually. Many women say they feel sensation in their feet and toes first, while others claim to feel intense pain in the area that has been cut. By the time sensation is felt in your stomach, you may be more conscious and need medication for the pain.

Waking up in a recovery room in pain, bewildered and perhaps confused or scared can be very discomforting. On the other hand, waking up to the sight of your baby and partner can create a feeling of safety for you and your baby and facilitate immediate bonding. Most hospitals will not allow anyone in the recovery room with you. You must request in advance that they be allowed to be with you. If more women speak out and ask for what they want, perhaps hospitals will continue to hear our requests and change their policies.

Some hospitals allow the partner in the operating room to hold the laboring mother's hand after an epidural anesthetic has been administered for a cesarean. The use of general anesthesia requires more involvement, and many hospitals do not allow "outsiders" in the operating room. When writing your birth plan, be sure to include all the possibilities. Request the presence of your loved ones while in recovery. Seeing a loving face and holding your new little baby are great for your morale and aid in grounding you and assisting in the mother-infant bonding which many women describe as difficult when they have not been allowed to see their baby for the first few hours after birth.

DEALING WITH PAIN

I remember being in my hospital room after my first cesarean. I was scared and in a tremendous amount of pain. Fortunately the staff of nurses were like angels from heaven. With each changing shift, they offered support for my fragile emotions, along with tricks for easing the pain.

- Patty, a 33-year-old mother, recalls, "After my cesarean I was so afraid to cough; I thought my stitches would burst open."
- Remembering her surgery, Barbara, age 28, and mother of cesarean-born Josh, says, "When I first passed gas, the whole staff went nuts. I don't know why they were so excited. I was so embarrassed!"
- Terry, who gave birth to her daughter by cesarean and had a VBAC with her son, adds, "I remember having to sneeze after April was born. I panicked because I knew I would rip everything open. I held on to the hand rails of the bed, bent my knees up, sneezed and then had excruciating pain for what seemed like ages."

After any form of major abdominal surgery, the fear of sneezing, coughing, laughing or having a bowel movement can be overwhelming. There is the underlying belief that any great effort of this kind will cause you to rip open. Rest assured you will not tear your

stitches apart. Putting one or two pillows over your incisi[
pressing firmly will greatly eliminate any undue pressure and
untary movement of your abdominal muscles. This is a simple
nique, but usually no one tells you this until after that first laugh or
sneeze, when you experience incredible pain and absolute fear your
insides will spill out all over the place with even the most minute
movement.

Your intestines also become paralyzed by the anesthesia and
surgery. Once your system begins to function again, any material
that was present in your intestinal tract before surgery creates gas and
causes your intestines to become distended. This can be extremely
painful. Therefore, the passing of gas and the first bowel movement
become major events after surgery. You can expect your doctor and
the entire nursing staff to celebrate wildly at these two events. Besides
any embarrassment you might have about these two very normal
bodily functions, it still may feel strange to have everyone in the maternity unit whoop and cheer as if it were Super Bowl Sunday!

With my first cesarean the nurses kept promising to give me ice
cream if I "did it." To facilitate a bowel movement, you might be offered medication to make it easier. I chose not to take any more medication than the one I needed for pain, as I did not want any more
drugs in my body or in my breast milk. I always recommend that
women do take pain medication if necessary. Take your medication
before the pain gets really bad. That way you can stay on top of the
situation, enabling yourself to function clearly. It is very difficult to
hold, breast-feed and care for a baby when your thoughts are clouded
by pain. As soon as you are able, stop taking your prescribed medication. Drink a lot of liquid to keep your body fluids flowing.

According to Hausknecht and Heilman (1991), exercise and early
ambulation reduce the possibility of pneumonia and phlebitis. Therefore I tried very hard to walk as much as my poor, wounded body
would allow. It is very important not to walk alone the first few days
after your surgery. The nurse, your partner or your support person
can steady you as you go. Additional medication in the form of
tablet or suppository is usually offered to stimulate your gastrointestinal tract. Walking will get your gastrointestinal tract flowing
again.

When I was a professional massage therapist, I learned a technique
to aid in the passing of gas. Take two fingers and place them on either side of your right shin bone, starting at the very bottom where
your leg bone joins your ankle bone. With the rounded tips of your

fingers, slowly move up toward the knee, firmly massaging each side of the bone as you inch your way up the leg. Hold firmly on any tender spot, then continue upward. When finished, do your other leg (or have someone do it for you). Repeating this technique two to three times on each leg a couple of times a day will stimulate your ascending colon and bring on that much awaited passing of gas quicker than anyone expected. Not only will everyone celebrate, but they will be awed at how you "did it " so fast! Silly as it may sound, this is a very important part of your recovery. This technique can also be used after any kind of abdominal surgery, and it even works wonders for constipation.

The hospital staff may ask you to do coughing and breathing exercises during your recovery. Deep breathing will help re-expand your lungs after anesthesia. Deep breathing also helps to rid your body of any residual anesthesia if a general anesthetic was administered. This particular breathing exercise may not be a comfortable experience, but the more you are able to practice this, with the aid of your hand over the incision as a splint or pillows pressed firmly against the incision, chances are you will speed up your recovery and get out of the hospital that much sooner.

EXERCISE

After surgery, you may feel bloated because of the effects of the medication in your body. In addition to walking, gentle exercises are a way to get your body to function again. The exercises can be as simple as rolling your ankles around in circles or making slightly more complicated movements. You can modify many of the simple yoga techniques you may have used prenatally while you are recovering in bed. Some beneficial exercise movements that you can do while lying in bed on your back are leg lifts, gently rocking your pelvis from side to side, wiggling your toes, ankle rolls, flexing your calves, and alternate leg raises. You can use pillows to prop up your knees, elevate your head and cushion your body wherever you feel you need extra support. Remember to take it easy; do not push yourself. Exercises you can do while sitting up in bed or on a chair are neck rolls, rolling your shoulders forward and back, arm circles, rotating your hands around, and gentle side bends. You can add any movement that feels good. Often women who were physically active during their pregnancy will feel inclined to get back in shape right away. Take it easy! Do not strain.

These gentle stretches and exercises are not meant to get your body back to your pre-pregnancy weight, but to allow you to function again so you can go home and begin your life as a family.

PSYCHOLOGICAL HEALING

Cesarean birth can leave emotional scars which last a long time and run very deep. There are many women who give birth to their babies without any long-lasting psychological trauma and they quickly settle down to the task of raising a new family. However, many women are affected in the way they feel about themselves and find bonding with their baby may be slower than they expected.

Jan was in recovery for three hours after the cesarean birth of her son. She did not see him until the next day, because the nurses kept him in the nursery so Jan could "get some rest." Bonding with her newborn was difficult, because she felt very guilty about not being with him immediately after he was pulled from her body. It was not until Jan began psychotherapy for postpartum depression that she began to understand how her own feelings of failure and sense of guilt caused her to be angry and impatient with her newborn son.

After hearing the stories of hundreds of women who have had cesarean sections, I have found that a planned cesarean can cause anxiety and depression. Yet, my personal work with many of these women has shown that the psychological implications of birth by major abdominal surgery that was not planned, anticipated or even remotely considered can be shocking to a woman. Waking up to the realization that her baby was "taken by cesarean" may cause a woman to blame herself, her baby or her doctor for the failure to birth vaginally.

The new mother needs an outlet to process some of her feelings immediately. This can be done with a care provider, therapist or friend who will take the time to listen. Do not assume what she might be feeling; ask her what she is experiencing within her heart. Typically, women who have had unplanned cesareans often feel victimized. Some say they feel like failures as women. They even express feelings that they have "hurt" their babies. Women need to be listened to so they can get in touch with their feelings.

The most common line of assistance offered by family and friends is "So you had a cesarean. Big deal. Thank goodness both you and the baby are healthy and alive." Other comments include, "But you have a beautiful, healthy baby; that's all that matters" and "At least you didn't have to feel any pain." I have heard women say over and over how much they hate these statements. Historically, many women have played the role of martyr, putting their babies first, sacrificing their own needs, not having clear boundaries and suppressing their true feelings. Giving birth is not just about having a baby. It is a peak experience in a woman's life in which she is affected on physiological, psychological and sociological levels. The realization that she has a beautiful, healthy baby does not always ease the feelings of guilt and shame that some women experience.

- Christina, a 22-year-old teacher, said, "I was so depressed after my cesarean section. I felt like I had failed the biggest test of my life: Womanhood."

- Joy was looking forward to a normal, uncomplicated hospital birth. For reasons she feels were unnecessary, she ended up with a cesarean section. Devastated, angry, and feeling sad that her husband could not participate in the actual birth, Joy became depressed. Her husband and her mother kept trying to reassure her that the baby was all that mattered. "The baby is beautiful, she's healthy and she has your eyes. Be grateful, pull yourself together and stop crying," her mother insisted.

- Emily was 25 when she had her first child. She reported, "Everyone kept telling me to be thankful that the baby was okay. I was so angry that the doctor had set me up for a cesarean. He gave me drugs without my permission, and then I was so numb I couldn't even push my baby out. They had to cut me open to get her out of me. It wasn't my fault. I wanted to push her out. They wouldn't let me."

It is important to believe that your body knows how to give birth naturally. In most cases, giving birth does not need to be a medical event. You must believe in yourself, your body and your ability to give birth. For many women, emotional clearing can help release conscious or unconscious fears or negativity. If you have given birth before, it is often very helpful to process your feelings from past birth experiences.

Anne-Marie kept trying to figure out what she did "wrong" during the medically oriented vaginal birth of her second child. "My first birth was a cesarean. Looking back, I think I just wasn't prepared. I tried to get ready for this birth, but I can't think of anything I could have done differently and the doctor did everything she could, but I'll tell you, this was not natural childbirth at all! Maybe I could have done something, anything else, but I can't figure it out." Anne-Marie could not think of anything that she or the medical staff did wrong. In this case, being able to talk and ask open-ended questions made her feel better. I have worked with many women who just needed to talk about their experience. They were not ready to look deeply into themselves to see how and whether they might have held themselves back, nor were they ready to question whether their care provider intervened unnecessarily. At this point of their recovery, they may be afraid of placing blame wrongly. Trying to find someone to blame will not solve anything. Being able to feel her emotions and speak what she believes to be her truth allows a woman to reclaim her own power and find her own strength. When a woman is feeling vulnerable it is important not to minimize her feelings. We need to listen and be supportive of her, so she can begin her own healing process.

With the availability of many forms of therapy and healing techniques such as positive affirmations, hypnosis, psychotherapy, rebirthing and support groups, a woman can dig deeply into her consciousness to clear out any negative ideas or thought patterns that may be lingering before or after giving birth. Many women I have spoken to insist they do not need therapy just to have a baby. We have all heard stories of friends who went into labor and joyously gave birth four hours later. What did *these* women do differently than the one half million women giving birth by unnecessary cesareans? Look at the excessive cesarean rate, the excessive number of women requesting cesarean births, the constant requests for epidural anesthesia to eliminate pain, the number of routine episiotomies being done, the number of complications that arise during a "normal" birth and the millions of women who "did not dilate," and ask yourself "what has happened to childbirth?"

Elena was having her first child late in life. As an executive in her own company, she was quite used to having things done her way. When she asked me to assist at her birth, she told me she wanted to avoid pain at all cost. An epidural was in order to eliminate any pain, and a "shot of something" in early labor to calm her nerves was on her agenda. She firmly stated "If I don't have to feel pain, why should I? I want the drugs."

After working closely with Elena for seven months, I watched her point of view transform. Like a seedling blossoming into a flower, Elena grew. She read about childbirth, studied all the new material on labor she could find, and opened her mind to a new way of thinking. After doing her homework she was determined to have her baby naturally, with little or no intervention and most certainly without the assistance of any kind of drug which could harm her baby or alter her own consciousness in any way. After convincing her family of her new-found beliefs and gaining the support of her husband, Elena was on her way to a wonderful birth experience.

Two weeks before her baby was due, Elena started having nightmares about the birth and her baby. Her dreams forced her to look at her fears, and she confided in me. In her nightmares, the baby would "get stuck coming out" or "look like a baboon" once it did come out. Elena was terrified that these thoughts would somehow stifle her labor. We scheduled two sessions in which I took Elena through a visualization process. In addition, we used affirmations so she could focus on positive thoughts and restore her belief in herself and the inherent wholeness of her unborn child. After each session, Elena reported that she felt better, stronger, and more trusting of herself. She remained strong and centered throughout her labor, and gave birth to a beautiful little boy after just twelve hours. Elena realized that it had been crucial for her to look closely at her fears and "let them go."

Eight years after the cesarean birth of her stillborn child, Helene, now 44 still suffers from occasional bouts of sadness and loss. She remembers people saying things like, "You'll have more children" and "You can get pregnant again soon, it's not so bad really." With great sadness, Helene said,

> The whole thing was horrible. I have a huge scar, and for what? I got nothing out of the deal. The nurses kept telling me to push harder. One nurse even said, "Push harder; don't you want to get this baby out alive?" I will never forget her words. Somehow that particular statement has stayed with me and added to my guilt. To top this whole thing off, I finally had a cesarean because my baby's head was deformed and too big for me to push through. Shouldn't they have known? Their bedside manner was so awful. I never did have another child, but I have that scar to remind me of the one I lost.

The International Cesarean Awareness Network (ICAN) offers support to women healing from any type of birth experience, as well as women preparing for future births. As the past president of the

Marin County chapter of ICAN for four and a half years, I have seen tremendous healing take place in women. The support, information and strength they gain from listening, talking and sharing with other women who have had cesareans are powerful. Women preparing for VBACs also receive support and empowerment from talking to other VBAC mothers. The women who have had repeat cesareans can come to the group and discuss their heartfelt emotions and birth experiences with other women who truly understand. Contact your local chapter of ICAN, P.O. Box 276, Clarks Summit, PA, (717) 585–ICAN.

Many women have been led to believe that their cesarean was necessary. They see the result of all the medical interventions as appropriate and continue to have faith in their doctors. While it is important to trust the person cutting open your belly, we, as birthing women, must assume some of the responsibility. Using the tools from Things You Can Do to Prevent an Unnecessary Cesarean (Appendix D at the back of the book), many unnecessary cesareans can be prevented.

When a woman is willing to look very deeply into her psyche, to honestly feel her full range of emotions, to assume responsibility for her upcoming birth experience, to trust her baby and her body to the extent of accepting whatever the outcome may be, to surrender to the greater powers that be, her birth experience can be more joyous and include less intervention.

When all is said and done, in many cases there are no answers or solutions. I have talked to women who thought they "did everything" yet still had complications and interventions they had not planned. We must make informed choices in childbirth, we must believe in our ability to give birth, and we must trust the baby's inherent desire to be born. No matter what the outcome, ultimately, we must accept and surrender to the process that is the miracle of birth.

Chapter 9

Healing Cesarean Section Trauma: A Transformational Ritual

Jeannine Parvati Baker

Jeannine Parvati Baker is the author of Prenatal Yoga and Natural Birth *(1974, 1986),* Hygieia: A Woman's Herbal *(1980), and* Conscious Conception: Elemental Journey Through the Labyrinth of Sexuality *(with Frederick Baker, 1986).*

She is a midwife, astrologer, herbalist, speaker, and the mother of six children, all born naturally. She is the director of Hygieia College, a mystery school in womancraft and lay midwifery. Along with her husband, she created the Six Directions Foundation, a non-profit educational and charitable corporation for healing sexuality, fertility, birth, family and our Earth. In 1993, she was nominated for the Woman of the Year Award by the International Biographical Centre, Cambridge, England, for her contribution to medicine.

Ms. Baker combines the ancient knowledge of midwifery, herbalism and ritual with modern psychology and current holistic knowledge as she brings wise-woman craft into a patriarchal, technocratic world. She is respected and admired for her gentleness, ancient wisdom and respect for all things great and small.

About her chapter she says: "In my Healing Cesarean Ritual, we come to realize the spiritual dimension of cesarean section which I term 'near-birth' as analogous to the near-death experience."

"Healing Cesarean Section Trauma" has also been published in The Goddess Celebrates *(1991).*

Birth is life's oldest ritual. Our society has lost most of the prenatal and postpartum supportive, preparatory and completion rituals for natural birth. Instead, we've replaced them with medical rituals which make natural birth much harder to experience. So it is to ritual that we turn to heal the trauma of surgical childbirth.

Delivery of babies by cesarean section surgery requires healing of the whole being, for both mother and baby, some time in the postpartum period. Ideally, the sooner a mother is willing to feel the pain of her loss and the insult upon her body, mind and soul, the better. However, we cannot push the river. When a mother is able to, she will experience her grief. Then it is appropriate to offer her the following ritual to assist in deeper healing and forgiving. Cesarean section can be revisioned to be an initiation into soul making, but, first she needs the release of the pain, the healing, and then she can achieve empowerment.

Cesarean section is a major psychological event of our times for mothers, and one which will continue to affect those involved for a long time. Better to integrate the experience and find the personal meaning, that is, the purpose, for the surgery. The assumption is that all things serve on this earth from the psycho-spiritual perspective. There is tremendous potential for deepening one's understanding of the meaning of life when the road of denial and pain has been cleared. As the Chinese say, "The bigger the front, the bigger the back." The more trauma involved, the greater the opportunity for transformational healing.

PREPARE THE CEREMONIAL SPACE

How the mother and baby enter the ritual space is extremely important. This is the central metaphor to be healed—leaving a space and entering new ground. The new ground is where the ritual takes place. It is prepared by cleaning and smudging the room—or circle of ground outside—where the healing ceremony will be held. Flowers, plants, crystals, rocks or cornmeal may be used to define a womb-like space just big enough for mother and newborn to sit in. Also include something to symbolize the placenta (a large, pancake shaped rock or a lumpy pillow) and two cords (or three if you had twins! Woven belts make good cords.) Choose something to symbolize your mate (marriage bundle, wedding memento, etc.). Also in this circle, place the mother's own personal medicine bundle, power objects, and one offering which she will either bury or burn. Possible offerings are a crystal (if she has chosen to bury it) or a poem or statement of what she is willing to let go of now if she has chosen to burn her offering. Finally a jar of earth (if the ceremony is to be held indoors) can be set in the sacred circle. First create this space before the actual entrance into the circle for ritual.

The mother next prepares herself by bathing and anointing her belly with special oil. She wears her ceremonial dress from pregnancy (or at least her favorite pregnancy dress). She puts her hair up. (If she has hair too short to put up, she wears a barrette or comb or ribbon.) The baby is prepared in the same way. If it is warm enough, let the baby be naked.

Now she is ready to begin. Mother and baby stand outside the circle and pray. First she lists all the things that she is grateful for, then she prays for guidance—that this ritual will be healing and all that passes will be pleasing unto her God-Us (Spirit). Then she carries the baby and steps into the circle, witness to her movement, thoughts and feelings. This is a particularly portentous moment. *How* she enters her sacred circle will reveal how to heal the trauma of cesarean birth.

Begin with centering and grounding rituals and any opening prayers, mudras, poses or practices which are already familiar. If the mother has not experienced ritual before, here is a suggested format:

> *Sing—*
> She's been waiting, waiting
> she's been waiting so long
> she's been waiting, waiting
> for Her children to remember
> to return[1]

> *Sing—*
> Where we sit is holy
> holy is the ground
> forest mountain river
> listen to this sound
> Great Spirit circling
> all around us[2]

After singing, the mother prays for what she wants, clearly, humbly and with affirmations of surrender to those forces much bigger than the desires of this person. Express gratitude again for being a mother, trusted to care for God's baby (babies) and pray to be worthy of this trust. Express love for the child in words and action. The baby may be still on her lap or may have crawled away by now so that there is a semi-permeable membrane around the sacred circle which lets babies in and out without altering the focus of the ceremony. It is fine for babies to move about while the mother remains planted on her new ground.

Next, give an offering to the four directions and mother earth. If the ceremony is outside, this is more powerful. Take some soil in hand during this offering to the mother earth and rub it on the mother's belly and the baby's belly (if accessible). Indoors, the small jar of earth is now used. While offering to the earth, focus on the scar from surgery. Visualize both the scar on the mother's belly and the mother earth as healed—no personal wound, no collective pollution. Lastly, give an offering to the Great Spirit, the Goddess, Heavenly Parents (or whomever or whatever the mother calls the Mystery). Light some incense, a candle (something of the fire element) to represent spirit. Let the flame and smoke carry the prayers heavenward.

The mother takes the placenta and ties the cord between it and her belly. If the baby is lying still, or within range of the circle, another cord is tied between the baby and the placenta.

Next, the mother listens to her heart. A drumbeat helps, but without the sound of the drum focusing on one's own heartbeat as a pulse, a rhythm, is sufficient.

Deeper into the inner sounds and rhythms the mother goes as she meditates on her experience of giving birth. The mother visualizes the labor and those choices which led her to being sectioned: not only her choices, but all her attendant's influences. One by one, she visualizes these decisions and forgives herself and any others involved in them. The mother focuses on the image of each birth attendant with compassion and understanding. To complete this part, the mother visualizes herself being cut open, delivered and sewn back up. She expresses any feelings she has, and forgives all, including herself. Now she takes her hair down. (Or takes out the ribbon or barrette.) Then the mother takes her offering and buries it, or if it is to be burned, throws it into the fire (wood stove, abalone shell, ashtray, etc.).

Place the placenta symbol on the mother's belly. Breathe deeply down to the rock or pillow. Visualize the intactness, integrity and strength of the womb and abdomen. Image a gold glow all around the incision scar. The wound reveals the cure. Invite a message from the old scar and listen for the word medicine which comes. Ponder these things in the mother's heart.

Now the mother takes her baby in her arms and begins the closure. She may sing her own heart song or any other which truly moves her toward love. A possible suggestion is:

We are sisters on a journey
shining in the sun
remembering the ancient ones
the women and the children
the women and the children[3]

Then comes the closing prayer. Include acknowledgment to one's personal expression of Spirit and speak gratefully to that force bigger than each of us for the healing ceremony. Gratitude for the mother's own birthmother is appropriate here—and all the foremothers who made her possible. Connecting through imagery with one's heritage of birthmothers is empowering.

Hopes for future freebirths may be shared aloud. And that which was learned in this cesarean will benefit subsequent deliveries. Stating precisely just what was gained from surgical childbirth continues the healing process. Remember, all things on earth serve.

Lastly, close the prayer by asking for the healing of our mother earth, that she will no longer be cut, poisoned, raped and her children torn from her body. (Cut—agribusiness, mining and deforestation; poisoned—chemicals, nuclear radiation and drug abuse; raped—treated like an inert, unfeeling being by men; tearing children from her body—extinction of animal and plant life and the senseless violence humans perpetrate on one another. These are symbolized in the cesarean section: the scalpel, the anesthesia, the abduction of the baby, and the severance of natural birth bonding.) The mother commits herself and her children to being change agents for evolution and vows to align her personal desires with the collective will of nature. She knows better than anyone else how our mother earth must feel and dedicates her family to making their earthwalk a gentle one.

Blessed Be, Amen and Ho!! It is done.

Mother and baby then leave the sacred circle, again watching closely for how one experiences leaving the holy place. Outside the circle, the mother unties the cords between herself, baby, and the placenta. The placenta is then buried (if a rock). If the placenta is represented by a pillow, this pillow is now to be used for ceremonies only.

Ceremonial feasting, or at least a warm drink to represent the first feeding, may follow. Focus on the nourishment which comes so gracefully from the mother, with joy and thanksgiving.

Birth is life's central mystery. No one can predict how a birth may manifest. Birth belongs to a people, not an individual person, and reflects the morphogenetic field (the invisible connections each human has with others of our species). Our dominant culture is anything but "natural," so it is no surprise that childbirth, even when the most natural life-style is lived by an individual family, sometimes needs intervention and medical assistance. This is not to say that any one mother's efforts to have a natural childbirth are futile. Just that birth is bigger than one's personal desires.

Healing the trauma of cesarean will facilitate deeper bonding to the baby, cleanse the old wounds and provide the new ground from which to transform a horrific experience into one of great power. Wherever there is fear, there is power. On a tissue level, old unexpressed pain constricts physiologic processes, such as childbirth. It is very natural to fear giving birth again after a cesarean. This inhibits the fullness of joy in sex, especially seminal intercourse. If one is afraid of the trauma of childbirth, there is an avoidance of the act which brings about pregnancy. So this ritual has the excellent side effect of also bringing more ecstasy into sexuality.

This ceremony is also invaluable preparation for a vaginal birth after cesarean (VBAC) for it "feeds the hungry ghosts" which clamor for attention in subsequent births. It is known among midwives that the birth(s) after a cesarean raises issues about the surgery—and the laboring mother must psychologically give vaginal birth to the surgically removed baby before she can deliver her present baby spontaneously. This ceremony clears the road for freebirth (natural birth without assistance). Whatever dynamic was involved in impeding the previous birth is still present until it is understood—is forgiven. The most effective tool to use during this healing process is prayer. For example, if a mother was sectioned at seven centimeters of cervical dilation because she was "stuck" or the baby was distressed, during her next labor, at seven centimeters, a prayer circle would be indicated if needed.

Share this ritual with all of our sisters who have been abused and/or rescued from the surgical knife. This ritual can be done privately—or for the community with extended family and friends sitting around the sacred circle to pray and sing along with the mother. However, if there are others present, it is extremely important that the mother perform all the actions of the ritual and is not a passive recipient of the healing process. She will be strengthened by the knowledge that she is the prime mover in healing herself—and that nobody else can do it for her. Having been sectioned, a woman retains an imprint of being rescued. As birth is an expression of all our lives, so each moment a mother can be aware of being co-creatrix rather than victim of her experiences is "preparation" for VBAC. This ritual therefore is most healing when initiated, practiced, and completed by the mother herself, rather than being done for or to her. This does not negate the need for community but refocuses responsibility where it can best bring about freebirth.

We can change the morphogenetic field and transform our culture into one which reveres the original ground of our being, mother's womb, and then, by extension, we can heal our earth by healing birth. Where do we begin? Right where we are. Healing one mother is healing our earth.

NOTES

1. Kealoha, A. (1989). *Songs of the Earth*. Sebastopol, CA: Celestial Arts. p. 160. Every effort was made to acknowledge the songwriters. If we overlooked any credit, please inform us so that we can rectify the omission.

2. Ibid., p. 179.

3. Ibid., p. 172.

Chapter 10

One Birth at a Time

Andrea Frank Henkart

When a woman says she is going to have "natural childbirth" or a VBAC after a previous cesarean or a medicated birth, I always ask what she is doing to make this birth different from the last one. Typical responses are, "Nothing really, except my doctor is supportive" or "Oh, I read a few books and I'm taking a childbirth refresher course."

Women preparing for childbirth should learn as much as they can about labor and delivery. Do not leave your destiny in the hands of doctors who are influenced by their own personal belief system, peer pressure, hospital procedure, medical protocol and time schedules. Studying birth to gain a better understanding of what your care provider is talking about is extremely important.

I have already mentioned many things that can facilitate natural childbirth or a VBAC, including preparing a birth plan, hiring a professional childbirth assistant, giving birth in the hospital with a different doctor or with a midwife who has hospital privileges, having a water birth or having your baby at home with the assistance of a midwife.

Various forms of emotional clearing work such as rebirthing, hypnosis, visualization, meditation, positive affirmations, prenatal exercise and an absolute belief in your body's ability to give birth naturally can all make a difference in the way you feel about yourself and your ability to give birth this time.

It is important to remember that you are not the same person this time around. You are already a mother and the previous child has prepared the way for this one to be born. You are older now; you are more experienced in life just by the nature of time passing.

It is also important to remember that this baby is different—this baby has her own birth script and is *not* the same as the last one. Your pregnancy may feel very different as well; you may be carrying differently, you may be more comfortable or uncomfortable. Whatever little difference you can find will help you to realize that *this will be a different birth*. Relax, gather your strength, and prepare for a new experience. Take active responsibility in this labor and delivery. Anything you and your birth assistants can do to assist you in moving from a "stuck" place into a less fearful, more powerful feeling within your body and mind will be beneficial.

Often, the memory of the last birth becomes hazy. By talking about your previous birth with your care provider or birth assistant you may remember some of the fears or difficulties you had last time and you can begin to look at ways to avoid those same obstacles during the next birth experience. Do not wait to be in labor to resolve your questions and concerns.

Some women review their previous medical records in preparation for a second birth. Be aware that medical records can be inaccurate. With my first birth, my records stated I birthed a boy. Actually, my husband held our daughter immediately after she was pulled from my body and stayed with her throughout her first two hours. Reviewing medical records can be scary. Reading about all the medication and interventions that were used which led to a cesarean or a medicated birth can be frightening and overwhelming. As new mothers tend to have "selective amnesia" (remembering only what they want) after giving birth, reviewing past birth records can help you to remember the details of your previous birth experience(s), and it can be a powerful way to avoid making the same mistake twice.

Couples counseling may help your partner better understand what this birth experience means to you. It is an opportunity for both of you to look at your fears and concerns and it provides you with a safe place to work out any unspoken feelings. Encourage your partner to read books appropriate for his or her level of participation in the labor and birth. This can create an understanding of the birth process and facilitate new communication skills.

Family support is also important to a woman going into labor, especially if she is having a VBAC. A woman can derive inner strength from a supportive partner, care provider and close influential family members. Of course, one can always change care providers, but changing partners and family is not always a choice! Avoiding unsupportive family members and friends with horror stories may actually be easier. Keep the lines of communication open while keeping out negative influences by letting well-meaning family and friends know that you only want positive input and reinforcement. You can keep family and friends informed from a distance if their understanding and acceptance are important to you. If you do want them more involved, have them meet your childbirth assistant, see the location where you will be giving birth, and read some of the material that helped you develop your philosophy and approach toward labor and delivery. Encourage support "your way."

The importance of good prenatal nutrition has been stressed in numerous books and magazines. However, according to the stories I have heard from some women, their doctors have shown concern over "too much" weight gain and advised low-to-moderate caloric intake. Lorraine told me her doctor *allowed* her to gain twenty-five pounds "or else." Linda was told she could gain no more than thirty pounds. She was constantly watching her weight throughout her pregnancy, because she did not want to disappoint her doctor! Our society is very weight conscious, and many pregnant women think they look fat, while in other cultures, a pregnant woman is honored, respected and considered beautiful. It is important to eat well and gain weight according to the needs of your body and your baby.

If you are pregnant and hungry, *eat*! Increase your caloric intake by five hundred calories daily, avoiding "empty" calories. Eat five to six small meals a day instead of three big ones. Listen to your body and your baby, and eat healthy food. Avoid highly processed and junk food. Drink sugarless juice and lots of water. Stay away from unhealthy cravings. Cravings are just the body's and baby's way of letting you know that you are in need of certain vitamins or minerals. If you look at all the foods you crave, often you will find a vitamin or mineral that each food item has in common. Eat whole, natural foods that are rich in iron, minerals, vitamin C and complex carbohydrates. Become aware of your body's needs on a very deep level. Remember, all the food, thoughts and energy you put into your pregnant body feed your growing baby.

Stoppard (1993) says, "Your baby's bones begin to form between weeks four and six, so it's absolutely crucial that your intake of calcium be high prior to pregnancy and that it remain high for the rest of pregnancy." Calcium-rich foods include fresh leafy green vegetables, soy products and broccoli. There is a theory that a diet containing too many dairy products may produce not only excess mucus for you and your baby, but a larger head that may be more difficult to push out. Taryn, a doctor's wife found truth in this theory. Her first son was born at home and weighed over nine pounds. Taryn recalls all the dairy products she ate while carrying him: "I ate so much ice cream and cheese while I was pregnant with Marc, but never attributed his size to the type of food I ate." Three years later, Taryn gave birth to her second child at home. "I was a complete vegetarian this time. I ate virtually no dairy products and when I did it was low-fat. I pushed my baby out with hardly any effort at all!"

While in labor you can facilitate natural childbirth, a VBAC, or prevent a cesarean section by staying well hydrated and well nourished. In other cultures, women in labor are encouraged to eat and drink, yet our culture often insists on nearly starving women in labor. Replacing fluids by drinking sugarless juice or water will eliminate the need for intravenous fluid for nourishment. It is harder to move around and remain ambulatory when hooked up to needles and tubes that can travel only a limited distance.

Gail asked me to assist at the birth of her second child. Her first son was born by cesarean and she wanted to have a vaginal birth this time. Gail decided prenatally that she did not want to be hooked up to tubes, machines or anything mechanical that would take away from the "natural" aspect of this birth. She labored at home for quite a long time with her husband by her side, moving and moaning to the beat of her labor. Gail casually decided when it was time to leave for the hospital, allowing for the forty five minute drive. Her husband, David, drove while I sat in the back seat with her. Gail laid her head in my lap and I stroked her hair while she labored. When we arrived at the hospital, Gail decided it was too soon to check in. She and her husband strolled around the parking lot. As her contractions intensified, she would lean on David and moan deeply like a wolf howling in the wind. Gail decided when it was time to enter the hospital. As she was shown to her room, the nurse handed her a hospital gown. When she put on an oversized tee shirt instead, the nurse told her it might get all messy and bloody. "That's why I brought an old one" Gail replied. She also refused the obligatory fifteen minute hookup to the fetal monitor. "No one ever gets away with that one" the nurse firmly told her. Gail reassured the nurse that her baby was doing just fine and suggested she look at the birth plan in her file that her obstetrician signed. "Well, we have to put in a heparin lock" I remember the exasperated nurse blurting out. Gail politely informed her that she would not allow anyone to put an intravenous tube into her arm to use "just in case" she needed an IV. Gail was polite, she was firm and she was in heavy labor. The nurse stormed out. I closed the door behind her. We were left alone for what seemed like a very long time. Gail was free to move as she pleased, and changed positions frequently. She rocked, she walked, she leaned and she swayed. She never laid down on the bed. When the doctor walked in, Gail was squatting next to the bed. The doctor said, "I need to check you, but I can't do it from that position." Gail fended the doctor off for another thirty minutes by claiming strong contractions each time the doctor tried to check her. The doctor was surprised that everyone in the room was so calm and that we had everything under control. She said she had never seen anything like it before. As the doctor was leaving the room, she asked me to promise to call her when Gail was ready to push. I agreed as I continued to reassure Gail that this baby would be born as planned. Gail moved around the room, changing positions often and making deep, guttural sounds. She suddenly told me that many of her contractions were "pushing contractions" and she had been pushing for quite some time. "My baby is coming out" she whispered to me. As the doctor rushed in she saw Gail squatting next to the bed with David and me at her side. "I'm not comfortable with you birthing your baby on the floor, I've given you complete freedom up to now. Will you get on the bed to push your baby out?" the doctor pleaded. Gail climbed up on the bed, gave two very strong pushes and gave birth vaginally to another son. As Gail and her husband embraced each other and the new baby, Gail looked over at me. As she gazed into my eyes she said "Thank you for believing in me."

While in labor, body positioning is vital. Walking, rocking, leaning and kneeling are just a few positions that can facilitate the progression of labor. Remaining free of tension and significantly increasing the ability of gravity to work by squatting, sitting or standing help the fetus drop down into the pelvis, increase the pelvic opening and take pressure off the major blood vessel of the uterus, the vena cava. If all this moving around causes labor to progress normally, then obviously the risk of cesarean section is minimized.

According to Cohen and Estner (1983), the lithotomy position, where a woman remains lying flat on her back, is said to have come out of a time when Louis XIV wanted to watch his mistress give birth to their child. While she labored in the next room, he is said to have sat in a chair, peeking through curtains. While she was lying flat on her back, she was positioned so that he could witness the emergence of their child. The local peasants were so enamored of this woman that they wanted to emulate everything she did, including lying flat while giving birth!

Modern day hospitals with their advanced technology do not always encourage body positioning to facilitate labor. Yet, as shown by Stoppard (1993), standing during labor increases the intensity of the contractions, while decreasing the pain. In addition, Stoppard shows that when a woman is supported in an upright position or a supported squat position, the duration of labor is significantly shortened because it is "more mechanically efficient" than lying down.

If you are hooked up to various machines, it becomes even more difficult to move around. Kitzinger (1993) says,

> It was not till the end of the eighteenth century in Europe that women began to lie down to give birth. Before that time they had walked around during much of labor and used labor stools or sat up in bed or on a chair. Birth stools were designed like horseshoes, with the open part at the front, were low on the ground so that the woman squatted, and sometimes provided support for her lower back as well as handgrips. As a result she was in a physiologically excellent position.

You can disconnect from the IV and fetal monitor and go sit on the toilet. Used like a birthing stool, the toilet allows you to remain sitting up while the force of gravity brings your baby down. Birthing chairs are used throughout Holland; in hospitals and homes by midwives who are the primary care providers for labor and delivery. More than forty percent of women in the Netherlands have their babies at home and the cesarean section rate is below seven percent (Gabay and Wolfe, 1994)!

In "Ode to the Toilet Seat" Sears and Sears (1994, p. 192) call the toilet seat a "natural labor throne." They also say that Michael Rosenthal an obstetrician in California calls the toilet a "self-cleaning, porcelain birthing chair." While sitting on the "throne" a woman in labor can find both solitude and a seat at the correct height for the semi-squatting position. "A proven recipe for better birth."

Avoiding excessive medication may greatly benefit the progress of labor. One intervention often leads to another, creating a domino effect. Lumbar epidural anesthesia, or "an epidural" as it is commonly called, is requested by many women to avoid pain. Kitzinger (1993) shows how a local anesthetic is injected into the space between part of the spinal cord and the dura, the outer membrane around the spinal cord. According to Hausknecht and Heilman (1991), contrary to what most doctors tell women in labor, the drug injected into the spine *does* cross the placenta. They go on to say, "The drug often interferes with the patterns of normal labor, sometimes slowing the contractions down to the point where you require yet another drug, oxytocin, to stimulate them artificially" (p. 198). The epidural effects on the baby revolve primarily around maternal hypotension (lowered blood pressure), and can result in reduced circulation which may lead to fetal depression or a "sleepy" baby. Stoppard (1993) has shown that epidurals can also cause side effects such as nausea, vomiting, hallucinations and shivering. Smith (1984) has shown that epidural anesthesia can also cause cardiac arrest.

In the article, "The Duping of America's Childbearing Women" (1990), Zorn discusses the excessive use of epidural anesthesia. Epidurals supposedly kill pain so that a woman does not feel the process of her cervix dilating, her baby descending into the birth canal and her new child emerging. It allows a woman to dissociate herself from the experience and eliminates her ability to remain upright and walk about during labor, not to mention the many side effects and complications associated with epidural anesthesia. A woman planning a VBAC may fear getting "stuck" exactly where she was stuck the last time she was in labor. She may not need an epidural or other drugs to get her through it, but may just need extra support and encouragement while giving birth.

Talking to other women who have had VBACs and listening to what they did differently the second time around may help a woman gain perspective and insight. Consumer groups such as Cesarean Support, Education, and Concern (C/SEC) and the International Cesarean Awareness Network (ICAN) provide a forum for ideas, knowledge, insight and emotional support to the thousands of women healing from past birth experiences and others fervently preparing for non-interventive births.

Obviously there are certain indications when a cesarean section is necessary. In fact, when it *is* necessary it can be a life saving technique for both mother and baby. The old adage "once a cesarean, always a cesarean" was declared "an outmoded dictum" by the president of the American College of Obstetrics and Gynecology (ACOG) in 1984. According to VanTuinen and Wolfe (1992), ACOG also said in

October 1988 that "VBAC should be recommended as routine practice when safe to do so" (p. ii).

If for some medical reason your planned VBAC or natural birth
turns into a drugged, medicated or surgical birth, you *can* recover
feeling good about yourself, your baby and your experience. I have
often heard women say, "This time I *really* gave it my all." I am reminded of the advice found in a Chinese fortune cookie, "There are
no failures, only lessons." This concept gives women permission to
accept life's experiences in a very positive way. We need to find ways
to be accepting of ourselves and our experiences and gain insight
into what lessons we need to learn in life.

Having a baby usually brings hope, excitement and great expectations. On the other hand, it is important for all pregnant women to
remember that there are no guaranteed outcomes. The possibility of
a medicated birth or a cesarean section cannot always be ruled out.
An unspoken fear that often lurks deep below the surface is the possibility of losing the baby. Ruth told me, "I had a dream that the
baby was born looking like a gorilla, then she died. I was so frightened." Shawna said, "In my dream my baby was born a rabbit.
When I looked at him, he just hopped away!" Margaret sadly told
her story, "My birth was beautiful. I was calm, the doctor was supportive, but the baby died the moment he was born. I'm so scared to
give birth now. I want to keep this baby inside me forever, at least I
know he is alive now."

Even though I encourage women to think positively, it is equally
important to acknowledge and talk about your feelings; do not sup-
press your fears. Preparing for all the possibilities that labor, delivery
and parenting may bring will give you the opportunity to find out
what resources are available. Once you know who would support
you in your grief or shock and how you might handle the situation
should it even arise, you can dispel any unconscious fear that may be
lurking around in your subconscious. Let go of your fears and go on
with the process of preparing for life!

The joy that a mother feels after giving birth on her own is a most
rewarding blessing. Recovery from a non-interventive vaginal birth is
much easier and faster than from major abdominal birth surgery.
The mother is elated and full of renewed energy, her partner is joyous at their shared success and the baby rests lovingly and safely in
mother's arms.

For years, fathers were not allowed in the delivery room, and
birthing rooms were nonexistent. Women changed that by speaking

up. As many women begin to switch to hospitals that will provide them with what they need, other hospitals are slowly changing their ways and following suit. Giving birth should be a labor of love. Speak up for yourself and for what you believe in. Communicating your needs and desires to your care provider is the most important thing you can do to avoid an unnecessary cesarean section or medicated birth. We deserve to be heard and respected as birthing women in charge of our bodies and our babies.

Chapter 11

The Husband's Role in Pregnancy
John Gray

John Gray, Ph.D., is The New York Times *best-selling author of* Men Are from Mars, Women Are from Venus *(published in 26 different languages) and* What Your Mother Couldn't Tell You and Your Father Didn't Know. *He is recognized internationally as a leader in the field of relationships and personal growth. For over 20 years he has conducted public and private seminars to enrich the quality of relationships and improve communication between partners. His unique focus is assisting men and women in understanding, respecting and appreciating their differences. Dr. Gray is known for his humor, compassion and simple wisdom that can only result from being an example of what he teaches. In his highly acclaimed weekend seminars for singles, couples and families, he entertains and inspires his audiences with practical insights and easy-to-use techniques for immediately enriching their relationships. Over 50,000 people have participated in his seminars in over 20 major cities.*

The author of What You Feel You Can Heal *and* Men, Women and Relationships: Making Peace with the Opposite Sex, *he has been a frequent guest of ABC, NBC, CBS television and radio including Larry King, with highly rated appearances on Oprah Winfrey and Phil Donohue.*

Dr. Gray assisted his wife through the vaginal birth of their daughter after her two previous cesarean sections. In his chapter he writes with compassion and understanding of women and men as he offers tools for greater love, trust and communication in pregnancy and labor.

Women today are more independent and self-sufficient than at any other time in history. This new-found freedom is a source of confidence and self-esteem. In contrast, however, being pregnant and giving birth has put them in a very vulnerable and dependent situation and can have a devastating effect on how they feel about themselves. It is a time when they need their partner's love and support most.

It is difficult for a strong woman to be in a role which by nature requires so much dependency. Emotionally she is not equipped to feel good about herself while being so dependent on her partner for support. Society is telling her she is desirable only when she is competent and organized. Suddenly, she finds herself changing: sinking into the confusion and insecurity of pregnancy.

Nature demands these changes. Her body changes, her mind changes and emotions take on a life of their own. Suddenly the work of creating a baby takes over and she cannot focus on business as usual. Thoughts do not follow the usual logical patterns. Powerful desires and urges are no longer neatly explained by reason. Emotional needs suddenly surge. All these changes take a toll on her self-esteem.

Although men do not realize it, pregnancy is a time when a woman needs her partner's support more than ever. In my relationship seminars, I always take new fathers aside and tell them this is the most important time in their marriage. She needs him more than she can ever put into words. If he can be there for her at this time she will be grateful to him forever.

Men are sometimes concerned that if they give a lot more of themselves during the pregnancy, this behavior will always be expected of them. This thinking may hold a man back from wanting to do everything to make his partner happy and fulfill her every wish, even if it makes his life uncomfortable.

I assure men that it is only for nine months and then things can return to normal. I suggest that during this time a man devote himself to his wife more intensely than during the courting phase of the relationship. Men have an amazing ability to do a job which requires sacrifice as long as they know there is a time limit. By remembering that it is only nine months, a man can make the necessary adjustments and changes. Not only will the relationship thrive for years after, but your new baby will be much happier. The happier the mother can feel during pregnancy, the happier the baby can be.

While I recommend that men bend over backward to offer their support, it is still not enough to ensure the best experience of pregnancy. Women need to understand that men cannot anticipate their every wish and need. Even though a man loves you he will not automatically know what you need. In many cases, to get what you need you must be specific and ask for it. "If you don't ask, you probably won't get."

The secrets of asking a man for support are more fully explained in my book, *Men Are from Mars, Women Are from Venus* (1992). The most important skill in asking for what you want is to be brief (Do not nag). You do not have to justify your requests with a list of reasons for asking. Just ask and be direct. You are entitled. You are pregnant and that is reason enough.

If you detect resistance to fulfill your requests, do not stop asking. Even if he is willing to support you, he may feel resistant. This is because he does not know for sure that what he is being asked is necessary. Repeatedly appreciating his efforts will decrease this resistance.

Many women are afraid to ask for too much because they are afraid men will resent them after a while. This will not happen as long as they feel appreciated for the ways in which they have given support. They may resist in the beginning but are happy to give when they feel needed.

The biggest mistake a woman can make is to assume that if her man loves her, he will know what to do and will offer his support. This is not true. At this time more than at any other he may just not know what to do, and for this reason he may even appear to withdraw. He withdraws not because he is mad or indifferent to her needs, but because he does not know what is required of him. He does not know what she needs. He needs a "job description." To make matters worse, many strong women do not really know what they need at these times either! They are so used to being independent that they do not understand or recognize their emotional needs. Generally the only way for women to discover their needs is to have the opportunity and safety to express and explore their feelings.

During pregnancy, a woman's emotional needs become stronger. Listed here are four of the most prevalent emotional needs that women may have. This list can be used by men to identify those emotional needs and to assist women in identifying their needs so they can ask for what they want. Women should not expect their partners to remember automatically what is on their list.

THE FOUR T's

1. *Touch*. A woman needs lots of touch and affection. She needs to be touched in an affectionate and non-sexual way ten to twenty separate times a day. Many men do not touch their wives with affection unless they are in the mood for having sex. This can make a

woman feel she is only loved when he wants sex, and she may begin to feel like a sex object. To counter this tendency, and to fulfill her valid need for touch-interaction, gently touch and stroke her, or gently scratch her back. She will feel greatly comforted and assured that she is desirable and loved. From time to time, offer to give her a foot, neck or hand massage. Start and end each day with a warm and loving hug.

2. *Talk*. Women need to talk more than men do. Many men think something is wrong with a woman when she wants to talk more than he does. This basic confusion can be easily dispelled by remembering that men and women are different. When women are upset or stressed, they talk to feel better. When men are upset or stressed, they stop talking and cool off.

It is important for women not to misinterpret men as uncaring when they do not want to talk as much. Sometimes a man needs to pull away from his relationship in order to come closer again later. At such times he may seem distant or indifferent to her. Simply ignore him at these times. Give him some space and do not try to get him to talk. After some time he will seem more available. When he has come out of his "cave," then he will be willing to hear you talk.

But do not try to get *him* to talk; instead, ask him to listen. Say, "I'm so glad you are here. Would you listen to me for about five minutes? I'll feel so much better, you don't have to say anything." Telling him that he does not have to say anything is a job description. He can now listen to you without feeling obligated to "fix" you or "solve your problem."

To support a woman through pregnancy, a man should remember that listening to her talk is probably the greatest gift he can give her. Although it is difficult and frustrating at times, it *is* the greatest gift.

The reason it is so hard for men to listen is that they instinctively listen for a logical flow. When women talk in order to relax and feel intimate in their relationships, they tend to speak in a non-logical manner. At such times they are not limited by logic.

A woman's nature is to wander through her thoughts and feelings in a process of self-discovery. A man is looking for the point and she may not have one yet. He must practice not interrupting her flow with solutions to make her feel better. Practice giving her some empathy; that is generally what she needs.

3. *Trust*. A woman needs to feel safe and protected. The last thing she should have to worry about in this emotional time is hurting her partner's feelings and angering him. Although many books talk

about sharing and expressing feelings, I strongly urge the man to contain his negative feelings and definitely not to become frustrated or angry with his partner. It is alright for her to lose her temper, as long as he can keep his.

If he does start to lose his temper and get angry, then he should hold on and calmly say, "I want to understand what you are going through, but I need to think about what you have said and then we can talk more." Take a time-out to think things through and calm down. There is *no* good reason to dump your angry feelings on her. Be a harbor of safety for her.

On the other hand, let her know that it is alright for *her* to be angry and to express her feelings. This reassurance will help her speak up and move quickly through upset feelings. Women move through their negative feelings best by having their partner listen. Arguing, particularly during pregnancy, is too threatening to allow trust to grow. Whenever a woman is upset and angry, one of the best things to say after listening without interruption is "You have a right to be angry."

Making it safe for a pregnant woman to express herself and her feelings without having to be logical and rational at all times will not only nurture a great relationship but ensure an easier delivery. By getting out of the logical and rational side of her intelligence, she can freely let go and surrender to the wisdom of childbirth which is contained in her body and unconscious mind. Childbirth is an automatic process as long as the logical and controlling mind can stay out of the way. An understanding and patient partner dramatically increases a woman's ability to let go, and this in turn allows the birth process to occur with ease.

4. *Time.* Women need to be reassured that they are cherished *every* day. When a man shares his personal time with her, it says to her that she is special and loved. It is not enough for him to devote himself to her well-being by going to work, working long hours, or making money. She also needs to experience him toiling in front of her and for her. On an emotional level it does very little for her when he is serving others at work. While paying the bills is essential, it does not give her the emotional reassurance she now needs more than ever.

The solution to this problem is to create a little time each day when you are attentive to her every need. I suggest that you devote the first twenty minutes after work solely to her. Pretend that she is your most important client and give her the same quality attention that you would give to your client. As soon as you are both home from work, let this special time begin. Do not let anything come before her. Placing her first will make her feel loved and cherished. Otherwise she will begin to feel neglected and ignored.

During this time, look at her a lot. When she speaks, always look in her direction. Occasionally touch her and at least once, give her a hug. Offer to do little things for her, but, most important, ask her questions about her day. Show her that you are genuinely interested and that you care. Ask her how she is feeling and occasionally ask whether there is anything you could do for her. Compliment her on her appearance again and again with little comments like "Your eyes are sparkling; you look great." Do not become critical of her if she is upset or negative. Instead, become more understanding and empathetic.

PREGNANCY AND YOUR RELATIONSHIP

Pregnancy is a psychologically confusing time and women need lots of *emotional* support during the entire process. By reviewing the list and focusing on "The Four T's," it can and will be an easier process.

A man also needs support at this time, but in a different way. He needs acknowledgment and appreciation for *whatever* he does. He needs to be *told* he is appreciated; he needs to hear that you think he is doing a great job. He needs to know that you are glad to have his support.

As a pregnant woman, you may find yourself in a negative mood, or crying with no explanation for why you are feeling sad. By acknowledging that your unexplained feelings may be hard for your partner to understand and letting him know that you appreciate all he is doing, *you* can make *him* feel good.

When a woman forgets that her man is different from her, it is hard for her to feel loved when he does not offer to support her. Generally, if a man does not participate in the birth of their child, it is because he does not know what to do. Remembering that he is different makes it easier to realize that he may want to offer support but just does not quite know how. The best way for a woman to teach a man to support her is by asking for what she needs in a nondemanding way.

There may be times when he may appear passive or uninterested. This is not because he does not care, but because he does not feel worthy of her trust. He is not an expert at childbirth and can easily and even happily give up control to doctors and nurses. Unfortunately, the experts do not always know what is best. A man needs to know that his wife trusts him and that his opinions are important to her.

Certainly a husband cares more for his wife's well-being than any doctors or nurses could, but he does not have the knowledge or experience they have. For this reason, I strongly recommend that men participate in childbirth classes. I recommend that women read to them sections of books that reflect their ideas about birthing procedures. This way, at the time of birth when the experts come in with differing points of view, and his wife is feeling very tired and vulnerable, the man can stand firm for her wishes. Remember, the doctors do not always know the right answers and sometimes their suggestions are tainted by their busy schedules.

Hospitals, doctors, and nurses can be very intimidating. When hospital procedures, doctor's orders, and nurse's suggestions conflict with the laboring mother's wishes and needs, she may have little strength to stand up to them alone. She needs her partner to stand by her and not side with the authorities.

Always remember, the hospital, doctors and nurses work for you. You are paying their bills. This is your child and they cannot control you. Do not worry about making things inconvenient, or for asking for second and third opinions. Do not believe what they say if it conflicts with what you have learned before or what you feel in your heart.

Be prepared with the ammunition of knowledge and do not be intimidated. You would never go into a restaurant and simply take what they give you. Look at the menu and make sure you get what you have ordered.

Ideally in a marriage both partners will feel safe and comfortable in asking for and not demanding what they need. During pregnancy is a perfect time for women to practice asking for support, because this is when they need it most.

Through practicing "The Four T's: Touch, Talk, Trust and Time," the birth process will be easier and your baby will be healthier. In addition, the loving bond between mother and father is greatly affirmed and will be remembered for a lifetime.

Chapter 12

Birth Stories from around the World
Andrea Frank Henkart

Never doubt that a small group of thoughtful committed citizens
can change the world; indeed, it's the only thing that ever has.
Margaret Mead

A woman's birth experience is influenced by the messages she carries around in her head. Stories we were told as little girls and stories
we have heard from our friends, relatives, and mothers while growing up all contribute to the unconscious fears and doubts we bring
into our own birth experiences. Some women have hidden belief systems such as "I can't push my baby out" or "I'm afraid I'll die while
giving birth" or even "I don't want to give up being a little girl; now
I'll have to be a mother." These are unconscious beliefs that we may
harbor in the depths of our minds, and while in labor we may unconsciously call them forth.

In many cultures birth is considered a natural passage into womanhood. The messages handed down from generation to generation
allow a young girl to grow up with positive images of birth. When
she is ready to give birth to her own child, she approaches labor and
delivery with a complete sense of trust, pride and confidence.

I was fortunate enough to witness this kind of positive belief system at the birth of Gittel's son, her second vaginal birth. She and her
husband are Orthodox Jews. They devoutly honored their religious
laws, one of which prevented her rabbi husband from being at the
birth of their child. While I assisted at her hospital birth, her husband prayed in the waiting room. Gittel's birth experience was the

most exquisite I have ever seen. With a far-away look in her eyes, Gittel swayed back and forth like a feather floating in the breeze throughout her entire labor. It appeared as if she were dancing her baby out. Her complete trust in her body and in God allowed her to have a gentle, easy, almost "magical" birth. Without any intervention at all, including the obligatory use of the fetal monitor, Gittel pushed her son out in five pushes. When we discussed her birth a few weeks later, I asked her what made her birth stand out from all the others. With a very determined look in her eye, she explained that birth in her family is a natural event. Her mother gave birth easily, her sisters gave birth easily, even her mother-in-law believed in this "woman's art." She then told me, "My body was made to do this, and anyway God knows what He is doing."

Most American women take childbirth classes to learn to breathe during labor. I have yet to see a woman hold her breath while in labor! Pregnant women in Holland receive education and information from their midwives during prenatal visits; they do not attend childbirth education classes. During my personal communication with Astrid Linburg and Beatrice Smulders, both midwives in Holland, I learned that midwifery is the norm. Doctors see only patients who have complicated pregnancies, and midwives have full hospital privileges. Childbirth as a whole is looked upon as a normal, natural experience. Contrary to our cultural beliefs about childbirth in America, the Dutch women and men receive positive, healthy, non-threatening messages about birth from the time they are young children. In Holland the homebirth rate is approximately forty percent, the highest among all the industrial nations. While the United States has a twenty two to sixty three percent cesarean rate, Holland remains stable at seven percent. In addition, the Dutch claim the lowest infant and maternal mortality rate in the world; America ranks way behind in twelfth place.

Between 1987 and 1993, I interviewed over one hundred women, some who were mothers, others who had not yet had children. In the interview, I asked women from many countries around the world to tell me what kind of messages they received about childbirth while they were growing up. If they had given birth, I asked them to write about their experience(s). What I discovered was that the majority of women heard stories about childbirth that were unpleasant. After receiving a lifetime of negative input, only ten women reported having positive birth experiences, all the others experienced childbirth as fearful and painful with a sense of being out of control.

I sent questionnaires to a midwife in Holland, asking that she give the questionnaires to her clients. Asking to remain anonymous, she wrote,

> Thank you for your letter. . . . Sorry, but I can't help you because there are so little people who get a cesarean section. I think in our practice one or maybe two pregnant women in one year get a cesarean section, or vacuum extraction or forceps delivery. I think in USA there are more of these done. Nearly all the women are doing the delivery at home. They know it is the better way.

How many large obstetric practices in America can boast of just one or two cesarean, vacuum extraction or forceps deliveries in one entire year? What's more, how many of these same practices promote the idea of safe, gentle, easy, *natural* childbirth?

Brunella Innocenti writes from Italy,

> Remember that the Italian situation is very different from yours—because of socialized medicine, we get "free everything"—hospital, medicines and five months full salary (2 months before birth and 3 months after birth). But if you give birth at home, you have to pay for everything yourself. Not everybody can afford to do this, but even if you do have a birth at home, you still get the full five months of paid salary!

Innocenti goes on to translate an article written in the much respected Italian magazine *L'Espresso* (February 28, 1993). According to Innocenti, the overall cesarean rate in Italy is seventeen percent. However, the rate of cesarean births drops to ten percent in hospitals that are "well organized for a non-violent and natural childbirth." In hospitals "who care a lot for the economical part of their business, the cesarean rate is 40%!"

Here are some responses from around the globe:

ITALY

Grazia, 32, was told, "Childbirth is so painful, it feels like your stomach will explode." She experienced high blood pressure and had a cesarean section for the birth of her twins. Very matter-of-factly she says, "One of the twins was in the wrong position."

Brunella, 37, writes, "My first child was born in the hospital. All my life I was told 'Childbirth is so painful, you must go to the hospital; it's really a lot safer.' When I decided to have my second child born at home everyone kept telling me, 'You are crazy to want natural childbirth.' 'You're responsible for this baby. You'll be the guilty one should anything happen to the baby.' At first I was panicky, then I got better information and I felt confident in my choices."

Francesca, 47, says, "As a child growing up I was told that childbirth is very painful. I also heard that you just have to do it. I knew I would suffer a lot of pain, but it was for a wonderful purpose. I had a forceps delivery because the doctors said my uterus wouldn't let the baby pass through. [I wonder what position this woman was in while pushing?—Editor's note.] Someone told me once, 'Look at all the heads in a crowd; they have all been born through a woman's body.'"

Annalisa, 31, received mixed messages about childbirth. With both negative and positive input, she chose to have her child in the hospital. "I was told that natural childbirth is the best way of giving birth. I was also told that the hospital is the only safe place for a childbirth. My experience confirmed my old belief that it's better to put yourself in the hands of the specialist."

JAPAN

Itsumi, 38, received mostly negative messages about childbirth: "It is very painful . . . just like that your bite can break bamboo sticks." "It was very tough for the first one, but it will be easier after that." "Childbirth is a battle for a baby and mother." Itsumi gave birth to her son by cesarean section. "My hips did not open quick enough; I suffered for 24 hours." She says that the messages she received prenatally affected the way she gave birth because "I accept to have a baby as one of the natural things a woman has to do. It is very painful; I just have to suffer. My grandma did, and so did my mother. I did not think that I was different from them. I was excited to have the special experience that only women can have."

Debbie, 36, was afraid to give birth. All of her life she was told that contractions were "real long and real painful. I thought I might go through the same trouble and possibly pass out before I gave birth!"

Kumiko, 35, was told that giving birth is very hard, but worth it. "Some lady said, 'I loved it.' I wish I could get pregnant again." Kumiko realized that after talking to many women and hearing all of their stories, "I wouldn't know how it was going to be until I actually experienced giving birth. In this way, no one really influenced me. I knew it had to be my own experience."

PHILIPPINES

Uni, 28, grew up believing that childbirth was "not any big deal." She says, "I had a natural delivery. After 23 hours of labor, the nurse asked me to squat. Somehow that helped me, and I gave birth to a 6 lb. 11.5 oz. daughter."

Aida, 35, gave birth to three children by cesarean section. She remembers three outstanding messages she heard about childbirth:

1. They said that once you give birth, you as a new mother have paid what you owe to your mother.
2. There's a superstitious saying in my country that a pregnant woman should not wash her underwear and have it hanging outside to dry during nighttime. It's a bad omen. But only the elite can afford to have a washing machine and dryer.
3. You should not think of something ugly when you're pregnant, or else your baby might inherit the ugliness. Always stay away from people you don't like.

Aida continues,

I was 8 months pregnant when my obstetrician decided to perform a cesarean section on me. This was done because of high blood pressure, and to save my baby if things got bad. The baby was 4.14 lb. and had to be placed in an incubator for almost one month. She was our first baby and I was so scared. After two years, I had my second baby through cesarean with no complications. She was five pounds and healthy.

After another two years, I got my third baby. I went into labor during my eighth month of pregnancy. So my doctor rushed to perform the operation for the third time. This time it was critical for my baby for he was only two pounds and had heart problems. He survived only for seven days. After this traumatic experience, I was so afraid to get pregnant again. Five years later, I had my last baby who weighed 6 lb. 13 oz. and was full term. He was born with no complications at all.

I think cesareans are good because you don't go into labor; the pain and agony of waiting for regular birth can kill you. Anyway, in the Philippines, cesarean section is expensive. Only those who can afford to pay can avail of cesarean birth, because there is no insurance. It is better in America because you can have cesarean birth easy.

Elvie, 42, was born in the Philippines. Her two children were born by cesarean section in the United States. Her story is quite moving:

With my first child, I was not happy with what the doctor had explained to me the reason for doing such a thing. My mother was at my side, not knowing what to do and very scared and confused. I have realized after the fact, that this should not have happened. I felt deep in my heart that I was not allowed to labor long enough. The doctor was so hurried. My real doctor was out-of-town, so the on-call doctor had to do the delivery. It was late Friday afternoon when they said I had an inverted uterus. Being a first timer, I felt I had no reason to ask details. I strongly believe that it is real unfair that women are rolled into the operating room just for the convenience of the doctor and of course, for the cost! This is America . . . and perhaps there is no more sense or sensitivity about what real childbirth is all about!

My mother had seven children of her own. She told me "Childbirth is the most beautiful experience a woman can ever experience in her life. The pain is unexplainable, the suffering, the agony, it's unbearable. Yet when that beautiful human being is out of the woman's womb and is separated from the umbilical cord that had that long and direct connection with that being inside, *all the agony* with the sweat on her brow and all of her tears and screaming suddenly vanish. Everyone's experience varies, we are all different. But there is always that same beauty of seeing that very precious one come out of you." . . . My mother will never quite explain the experience of birth, yet she will always say it is beautiful . . . you have to feel it, suffer it, and bear everything laid upon you.

I wish I was left to experience the same kind of enduring pain my mother went through. My mother was with me when I gave birth, not understanding that I was cut, and that I was not allowed to let the Lord and nature take their course.

I am personally against C-section. Doctors (especially men) should not be allowed to deliver babies. It should be a midwife's job. I also firmly believe that unless it is a matter of life and death, this kind of elective surgery should be forbidden, absolutely.

Jeanne is Korean. She gave birth naturally to her daughter while living in Scotland. She was told six outstanding ideas that she will never forget.

1. Don't do it; the little buggers aren't worth it.
2. Just like sex, you just have to do it, no way to get around it.
3. You see this shriveled raisin-like baby and wonder to yourself, "Will this thing prove to be worth all this?"
4. I screamed like a banshee, cursing everyone in my family back to Eve.
5. Don't take any drugs; do it naturally. Otherwise you don't experience the birth.
6. It didn't hurt; the joy overwhelms the pain.

ENGLAND

I interviewed twenty young women of British nationality who were between the ages of 16 and 18.

Charlotte, 16, says, "From the television, I got that it is very special when you hold your child for the first time. I also saw on the television how some women have a very short and easy birth, while some can be in pain for hours and hours. My mother told me that she had terrible stretch marks from me and my sister." When I asked Charlotte how these ideas might affect her belief about childbirth and her potential ability to give birth, she responded, "I personally would like to be in a state of full awareness of what is going on when I give birth. I think it is important to hold your child as soon as possible after it is born. I would not like to be under any anesthetic because I want to take in the full effect of this special moment."

Yvonne is 18. Her mother told her, "My beautiful hourglass figure was transformed into a serious rectangle!" Another woman told her, "My breasts actually reached a decent size when I was pregnant." Yvonne also recalls being told how much pain she caused her mother. Yet, despite her images of body transformation and breast enlargement, she says, "I'd love a kid—natural childbirth, no drugs!"

Vicki, also 18 years old, remembers hearing about sagging breasts and stretch marks. She was also told, "You age ten years once you have children!" She says, "Some people say it's absolutely painful, but others say it's a wonderful experience. I am very confused about this. It is a bit offputting as people complain how painful it is to give birth, but I still think that the end product is worth the pain."

Despite hearing mixed messages such as "Childbirth is excruciatingly painful" and "Have nothing but natural childbirth," Christina, 18, says, "I'm frightened about stretch marks, sagging breasts and the pain, but I'll have a baby someday anyway. I'll do it naturally; that way my baby will be safe and I'll be able to have the experience of being a mother. I really want to have a child of my own to love."

Claire is 16. She can only recall hearing positive, happy images about childbirth. She says, "People's opinions wouldn't affect my beliefs about giving birth. I want children; pain is immaterial and forgettable. People have suffered for years; why try to stop the pain now?"

AMERICA

Karen has three children. While growing up, she was always told, "Giving birth is awful," "It hurts real bad," and "You shouldn't do this." She said that giving birth to her first child was very painful and that she did not really get very involved in the birth because she carried so many other people's negative attitudes with her. Her next two children were "very easy to deliver" because she was "experienced, in good shape, educated and aware of her options."

Gina is the mother of three beautiful children. Her mother was born at home in Sicily. When her mother gave birth in America, Gina was born by cesarean section. Gina says, "All my life I was told that I would have all my children by cesarean because I was petite like my mother. My mother also told me that having children ruins a woman's body for life. She also told me things like 'You should thank me every day for suffering so much to bring you into this world.' Other women told me that they wouldn't go through another pregnancy for a million dollars." Gina *is* petite, yet she was able to birth all of her children at home with the assistance of a midwife. When I asked her to explain the difference of her belief from the messages she heard, Gina replied, "I trust the miracle of birth."

Maria believes that birth is "very positive. It is important to prepare mentally and to trust the process and the body's ability to
have a baby. You have to trust the innate intelligence of your
body." Her personal beliefs emanate from solid family messages
about birth.

> I had three aunts in particular who I spent a lot of time with as
> I was growing up. My mom and my aunts never shared any
> negative stuff or horror stories about birth. They never tried to
> make any of us kids feel guilty for making them suffer or any-
> thing like that. My mom's recollection of her five births (six
> kids, I'm a twin) was always positive. She would say "It's no
> problem," "It goes fast," "You can do it; it's easy," "I love you
> kids." This all comes from a woman who was forced to keep
> her legs crossed during the pushing stage in her first birth be-
> cause her OB wasn't there yet!! But she never dramatized the in-
> cident. My mom is very supportive of home birth and my twin
> and I each had two children born at home.

Robin Lim, author of *After the Baby's Birth: A Women's Guide to
Wellness*, wrote to me from Bali. She briefly described the birth of
her fifth child:

> He was born in our little house in the village of Nyuh Kuning,
> Bali. Ibus (mothers) are supreme here, and as we live in a large
> extended Balinese family, we have many Ibus. They brought
> ceremonial offerings immediately after Wayan's birth. The ritu-
> als are still going on to welcome, protect and bless his life. The
> Balinese worship children (and old folks) as they believe they
> are closer to the Gods.

Robin remembers,

> My mother was from the Philippines. All of her five births were
> drugged births in U.S. Military hospitals. She felt dreadful
> about it. Her mother was a Filipino midwife; native plants, a
> knife and her hands were her only tools. My grandmother
> caught two generations of barrio children. She loved birth (she
> had ten of her own), and loved mothering, as I do. My mother
> describes mothering as a "bummer." Perhaps I purposely can't
> remember too many of my mother's messages about childbirth,

whereas those non-verbal messages my grandmother gave me are what I live by.

Giving birth is a significant life experience. For many, having a baby is linked to feelings of self-worth and identity as a woman. As our culture is besieged with a highly technological race to perfect birth, I can only hope that women maintain that natural childbirth is our birthright. We must teach our children that giving birth is a normal process in the cycle of life. We must teach them (and ourselves) that healthy pain is normal and helps us to grow stronger as human beings. As birthgivers, we must teach our sons and daughters to respect labor as the powerful birthforce of Creation. The way babies are born into this world, the way they are treated, and the messages that are handed down to them will affect the way they relate to the rest of their lives.

Chapter 13

A Balinese Cesarean Story
Robin Lim

Robin Lim is the author of After the Baby's Birth . . . A Woman's Way to Wellness *(1991), and* Birth . . . The Myths, the Facts, and the Rituals *(due 1995). She has written articles for* Mothering Magazine *and numerous newspapers and magazines. Ms. Lim lives in a small village in Bali with her husband and five of her seven children. She is on the advisory board for the non-profit organization Yayasan Ibu Sehat Bayi Sehat (Healthy Mother, Healthy Baby), and is an active midwife who is working to improve health care for women and children.*

Ms. Lim says, "My work in women's health takes me from hospital surgical rooms to the most intimate places of people's lives. I'm often paid in coconuts—though all my work is volunteer. The most common causes of death in Bali are complications from pregnancy and childbirth, with the two biggest killers being maternal hemorrhage and newborn apnea. It's time to do something about it."

This story was originally sent to me in the form of a personal letter from Ms. Lim. As I read about Dayu and her experience, I was deeply moved. It is from Ms. Lim's experience with childbirth and her gentle wisdom that she writes her chapter. Looking at childbirth and cesarean section from another culture gives insight into the "cesarean section madness" and the way many women all over the world so easily give their power and self-knowing away.

Dayu's hair flows down below her knees. She is twenty-seven years old and has a three and a half year old daughter, Putu. Dayu also has the biggest lateral cesarean scar I have ever seen. She never labored. She said, "The doctor told me the baby was too big." Putu was just over three kilos. Dayu and Budi want more children but Dayu is afraid of another operation. VBAC is unheard of in Bali.

The cesarean rate is increasing at an alarming rate *internationally*. After one year in Bali, I am appalled at the number of scars I have seen. Allopathic medicine (Western style) in developing countries is a frightening and powerful presence. Birth control devices and drugs are distributed widely, without any information regarding possible side-effects. United States drug companies dump untested and illegal devices here as well. This is all part of an effort to "control population." No thought is given to the health or well-being of the women or their children. They are, after all "brown" and of no consequence to American business interests!

The cost of cesarean births here in Bali is between one hundred forty thousand rupiahs ($70.00 U.S.) and three hundred thousand rupiahs ($150.00 U.S.). Natural childbirth costs approximately one-half of that amount. If you are white, a cesarean section now costs six million rupiah ($3,000.00 U.S.), twenty times the normal cost.

Midwifery is legal but is highly controlled by the government. *Bidans* (midwives) generally work in clinics or deliver at their own small birthing-house centers, they will make house-calls if asked. Midwives in Bali use a lot of Western medicine and distribute birth control devices. Generally, they do not practice very hygienically. For example, many do not wash their hands between patients. What's more, poor nutrition predisposes approximately eighty percent of Indonesian women to postpartum hemorrhage. There is virtually no prenatal care available and no chance for pregnant women to get the nutritional advice they need.

I've seen beautiful Asian women standing in the water at the river, badly scarred. Stitching here is not done artfully in layers, but straight in and deep. A few amount of stitches are used to close big wounds. There are usually three, very thick lateral scars, one for each child. The woman is told that three children is her limit, because the doctor has run out of places to cut! Is this how it is done in the West?

In all fairness, I've now seen two cases here in Bali in which cesarean birth saved lives. One quickly overlooks the primitive hospital conditions and practices when faced with a severe placenta previa, which threatens the lives of both mother and baby. In one instance, the condition was diagnosed by ultrasound in time to save both mother and baby. Good prenatal care alerted the parents to the danger and directly resulted in a happy outcome. In another case, the placenta did abrupt (peel away from the uterine wall) and the baby did not survive. Lack of adequate prenatal care resulted in loss of precious newborn life.

On the other hand, victims of cesarean section madnes[s] [In]donesia generally receive better postpartum care from their [__] than do most American women. This is the beautiful news about village life in Bali and their religion, Balinese Hinduism, which is the hub of *everything* here. In our village a new mother and her baby are served, honored and protected. Both men and women consider it a privilege to be of service.

Women who have had cesareans here do breast-feed. They consider it "abnormal" to bottle-feed a baby. However, giving birth in a hospital in Indonesia means that your baby will be given free samples of infant formula donated by giant Western corporations. This unethical practice continues even though in 1986, the United Nations proclaimed that giving free samples of infant formula to hospital and clinics in developing nations is against international law. After being bottle-fed formula while in the nursery, babies do not want to breast-feed. Indonesian women *expect* Western women to bottle-feed. They don't even dream of bottle-feeding as an option for their babies. They are always delighted when they meet a Western woman who is breast-feeding her infant. The Balinese worship children and old people, they believe in *Ibu Su-Su* (breast-milk), and also believe that mothers (Ibus) are supreme.

Indonesia needs well-trained midwives adept in the current protocols for safe natural delivery of babies, with a focus on non-intervention. Indonesia's maternal mortality rate has been estimated at seventy eight times higher than the average in developed nations. It is the highest in South East Asia. This high figure is a very conservative estimate, as eighty percent of the births take place in the homes, without benefit of a health provider. Therefore the majority of deaths are not reported. The infant mortality rate is so high that there is virtually no way to determine what it may be. Mismanagement of labor contributes to the extremely high rate of cesarean section and high risk delivery in the hospitals. A little knowledge has proven dangerous in the hands of well meaning bidans. Misinformation about the use of medical procedures sets the stage for standards of practice which are cruel and unnecessary, such as all first time mother's must have an episiotomy.

Indonesia, like the West, still has much growing to do in the field of obstetric medicine. It is a big job, but the bidans and doctors are eager to learn.

Chapter 14

Parenting the Precious Newborn
Andrea Frank Henkart

The body ownership we demand for ourselves, needs to be extended to the babies we bring into this world through the gentle birth process.

Marilyn Fayre Milos

The gentle birth movement began many years ago. With soft lighting, a minimal amount of noise and distraction, an untraumatized delivery, and gentle handling of the newborn, an environment of peace and serenity is created. Born into an atmosphere of love, the passion of creation is culminated. Those first moments of life are precious. A baby born into a loving, respectful environment will open her eyes, stretch out her arms and begin to discover the world around her.

Instead, most babies born in the hospital are shuffled down the assembly line of the system. The baby typically is whisked away from her mother, sometimes never even laying eyes on her. Then in the arms of a stranger, the baby is roughly wiped with (albeit soft) towels, then she is poked and prodded, pulled and stretched all for the sake of knowing her length and weight. Even though the father may be along for the ride, the baby, naked and alone, screams for (someone to protect her) dear life. Next, an ointment is automatically placed in her eyes. The baby is rendered temporarily blind. Try slathering ointment in both of your eyes and look at something you have never seen before. Try to make out details, colors, size. It can be alarming to have your vision blurred. A tiny, helpless baby who has never seen her parents, not to mention the bright lights of the nursery or intensive care unit, may be terrified to have these new sights turned into a messy blur. *The Amazing Newborn* (Klaus & Klaus, 1994) shows expressive photographs of attentive, alert babies just minutes old. "Their eyes are wide open, bright and shiny. Within the first hour of life, normal infants have a prolonged period of quiet alertness, averaging forty minutes, during which they look directly at their mother's and father's face and eyes" (p. 9). With their vision blurred by routine medication within minutes of birth, many babies and their parents miss out on these precious moments.

The baby is then subjected to a sharp jab of a needle pricking her, while a foreign substance, vitamin K, is injected into her pure little body. Sudden pain can lead to distrust! The vitamin K shot, routinely given in American hospitals without our permission, influences blood clotting. It was originally given to newborn boys to prevent hemorrhaging while circumcision was being performed. However, what most pediatricians neglect to tell the mother is that vitamin K is produced naturally by the body after the baby is born. Dr. Robert Mendelsohn links the vitamin K shot to newborn jaundice (1981), which requires more treatment and potential hazards to the baby.

"They say that a traumatic birth such as cesarean section, forceps or vacuum extraction warrants vitamin K to prevent a possible hemorrhage," said one obstetrician who wants to be unnamed. I asked him why so many doctors do not want their name in print. He replied, "It's strictly political. If my colleagues find out what I really think, I'll have nothing but trouble. We all have to conform to the standard of practice dictated by ACOG. If I didn't have to do all those things to the newborn, believe me, I wouldn't."

After more rough handling, pulling and probing, the newborn is wrapped tightly in a blanket and presented to her mother. Unable to handle all of the trauma after the birth, the baby often falls asleep. The new mother sees just a face, eyes closed, or a face staring out at her through smeary eyes. Anne said, "I had no idea I could unwrap my baby: I really wanted to see her tiny toes and fingers. It was two days later when a friend came to visit me in the hospital and told me that this was *my* baby, and I had every right to unwrap her and see her little body. That first skin to skin contact was a wonderful feeling for both of us."

Rob's wife gave birth to their first child, Samantha, in the hospital. Rob says,

> I refused to let them take my daughter away from us. I insisted they wait to weigh and measure her. She wasn't going anywhere! I unwrapped her, placed her against my skin and cuddled with my daughter. We formed an immediate bond that has lasted. The nurses were shocked. How could I expose her to my skin, and all those germs. Did they forget that it was partly my "germs" that created her? I never did let them take her away from us. We checked out AMA (Against Medical Advice). I signed a few forms and that was it!

Dr. John Gray (1992), *The New York Times* best-selling author of *Men Are from Mars, Women Are from Venus,* told me:

> When our daughter Lauren was born, they wanted to take her away from me and my wife to bathe her, weigh her and do tests on her. I insisted on holding my baby, carrying her and staying with her the entire time. Being with my new daughter through that ordeal was a very beautiful and bonding experience. Years later, she still delights in the story of how I carried her while she sucked on my finger.
>
> The nurses frowned at me and said I was going to spoil her. Certainly not all nurses are that insensitive and ignorant, but treatment like that does happen. Fortunately, I had been forewarned not to be intimidated by their "expertise."
>
> I would like to emphasize that there is no way to spoil a child with too much attention, holding, or feeding in the first two years. By giving to your child everything you can possibly give in those first two years, your child will feel that she is not powerless to get what she needs. More attention will not spoil your child, but instead will help your child to feel powerful and capable of getting what she needs in life.
>
> When your child cries, go to her, hold her, and attend to her needs. Sing to your child, talk to her, read to her, and love her. Attention, touch, love and food are the greatest needs of a child. When a child's needs are neglected in any way during this time, the child may develop feelings of powerlessness. That feeling of powerlessness tends to stay with them the rest of their life. Your child's birth is a powerful bonding time be-

tween parents and child. Plan it wisely (personal communication, 1994).

Norm's newborn son was hospitalized for three days after a home birth because of a respiratory problem. He and his wife took turns holding the baby for the entire three days.

> The birth went great. It was only four hours, intense and beautiful. But Cody was born blue because the cord was wrapped around his neck. He had so many things done to him in those first few moments of life. I just kept talking to him and letting him know that we loved him and that I wasn't going to let him check out. One of us always had at least one hand on Cody during every routine check that was done to him. Because of his problem, the doctor wanted to give him antibiotics to prevent any infection that might come up. I told him if an infection came up, we would talk about what he needed. I wasn't going to let them give him anything he didn't need. We still avoided eye drops and shots and all that stuff. But, boy did we have a lot of explaining to do and waivers to sign! We planned too long for this birth not to be just the way we wanted it to be. Cody's experience had nothing to do with the birth itself. It was partly his own experience he had to go through. But my wife and I stayed with him the whole time and stuck up for him. He's *our* son.

A gentle birth does not end as the baby emerges. It is just the beginning. Even if the birth did not turn out the way you dreamed it would, you are still the only one who can advocate for your newborn. She does not yet have a voice of her own. Start advocating for her now. As parents, we need all the practice we can get as our children grow into young adults who will need our support and need to know they can count on us. Cohen and Estner say, "Even when the baby is 'allowed' to be with you after the birth, many hospitals still view the baby as their possession. The time *will* come when hospitals will ask your permission whenever they touch your baby. They should be doing it *now*. They are holding your precious treasure, and should certainly have your consent before 'handling the goods'" (p. 198).

Know where your baby is going and what routine tests will be performed on her before she is whisked off to the nursery. You have the right to refuse any tests you feel are unnecessary by signing a waiver that releases the hospital and doctors from any liability, or you can insist that the tests be delayed. You must speak up for your newborn. If the baby does require emergency treatment or must go to the intensive care unit, stay involved. Know your rights. Do not give up your power as the parent(s). Your baby still needs your loving presence. Feel free to stay with your baby in the nursery, care for your baby and talk to her as much as you can.

Marie and her husband took turns holding their newborn while he was hospitalized for four days after his birth. They worked in shifts, insisting on changing his diapers, feeding him and participating in all of his treatment. He was constantly held, rocked and talked to by his mom or dad in those first, crucial days of life. She said, "That's my baby and I'm not letting him go anywhere without me."

While some babies do have health problems that warrant medical treatment, too many babies are diagnosed with the "threat of jaundice." A yellowish discoloration of the skin and eyes, jaundice is a result of excess bilirubin in the newborn's blood. Bilirubin is a yellow pigment which comes from the breakdown of the oxygen-carrying protein present in all red blood cells which commonly occurs after birth. Jaundice is almost always caused by an immaturity in the system which is slow to metabolize and excrete bilirubin. Kitzinger (1993) says, "If your baby looks beautifully suntanned as if just back from a cruise in the Bahamas, he or she has jaundice" (p. 335).

Half of all babies develop physiological jaundice. It becomes apparent by the second or third day of life and may last up to ten days. At that time, the excess red blood cells have been destroyed and the baby's liver has matured enough to deal with the excess bilirubin, which is broken down and excreted in the feces.

A jaundiced baby needs sunlight and frequent feedings. The full-spectrum light breaks down the bilirubin pigment in the skin and the nourishment stimulates the baby's digestive system.

After the cesarean birth of my second child, I told the hospital staff my son was to remain in my bed even if I was asleep. (Read *The Family Bed: An Age Old Concept in Childrearing* [1987] by Tine Thevinen if you have any fears about sleeping with or rolling over on your child.) The hospital staff was concerned my son's color "might" turn bad and that he would develop jaundice. They wanted to keep him in the nursery and bottle feed him all night long. Because my milk had not quite come in yet, the doctor felt this was a good precautionary measure and *insisted* I follow his advice. I decided to keep my baby safely by my side.

I did not want my baby drinking non-nutritive fluid in a bottle. Glucose does not contain the necessary protein that breast milk has. I trusted my intuition and knew my son was not going to show any symptoms other than this mild yellow coloring. I also knew that my colostrum (the condensed droplets that come out before the milk comes in) is full of protein and stimulates the baby's digestive tract. Once stimulated, the baby will pass meconium, the greenish black stool that is in his intestines. The meconium contains bilirubin, which can be reabsorbed into the body if not passed quickly. Nursing allows the baby to have the bowel movements his body needs. I actually woke my son every two hours during the night to make sure he had whatever fluid I could produce.

Cohen and Estner (1983) state, "Almost all newborns have some degree of jaundice; almost 60 percent of healthy, full-term babies show signs. Something that common must be normal and harmless; in fact it seems to be a natural part of the newborn's adjustment to life."

Because sunlight is known to break down bilirubin that has accumulated in the skin, I laid my son next to me, removed his clothes and placed diapers under his bottom. Fortunately, my hospital bed was next to a window. When the minimal sunlight filtered through the small window, my son's body was exposed to natural sunlight. Mother-intervention proved to be best in his particular case.

There are several different causes and types of jaundice. Pitocin, morphine and vitamin K are known to interfere with the baby's ability to handle bilirubin. Differences in blood type between mother and baby can create an incompatibility that may need to be treated by a blood transfusion. Kernicterus is the yellow staining and damage of brain and nerve tissues by grossly excessive levels of bilirubin. Jaundice is just one of many issues a newborn may face. Know your options. Trust your intuition, hold your baby close and nurse often. Do not be duped by doctors insisting on precautionary measures that are not really necessary. Being informed and making conscious choices allows you to maintain your power and work with your medical team. Tender, loving care is an important prescription for the health of your baby.

Another important aspect of baby health is breast-feeding. It is important to note that even if your milk has not come in yet, babies need to suck. They feel secure in their mother's arms (it helps if the mother feels secure and loving too). Your baby was secure in your belly for nine months; he is used to hearing your voice, feeling you from the inside and feeling your heart beat and your body breathe. Hold your baby close to your breast and convey your love to this innocent being. Your baby needs you now. The newborn stage passes in a fleeting moment of time, so do not waste a minute.

Some physicians, some husbands and even some mothers feel threatened or puzzled by the intensity of the nursing relationship. It is one of great intimacy and should be treated with respect and great reverence. It is a miracle to watch a baby grow just from the food a mother produces from her own body. Babies do not usually need supplementation or a bottle of water. They need the warmth and love and milk from their very own mother, not from a can of formula or from a cow. The more frequently the baby nurses, the more milk you will have. If you start your baby on a bottle, the baby will often prefer the bottle simply because she does not have to wait for a "let-down reflex" to bring on the flow of food. Someone once said, "Breast is best!"

Some women say they want to give their baby a bottle because that way, "Daddy can participate in feeding the baby too." Fathers participate in the creation of the baby, they can participate during the birth, they can be loving, supportive husbands and wonderful fathers. But they cannot breast-feed a baby; that is a job for mother.

Miriam and Dan prepared well for the hospital birth of their third child. Miriam hired a doctor who believed in the miracle of birth, and she created a birth plan with her birth assistant. Her birth was "gentle, easy and joyful. I love having babies," she said, as she held her new son in her arms. They checked out of the hospital five hours after the baby was born. Miriam said that as she nursed each new baby, "Dan would sit with me whenever he was around and talk to the baby. Sometimes he would hum or sing a little song. It was so sweet. He never felt competitive with any of our children. We have such a close knit family, I'm really lucky." On the other hand, Matthew vehemently told his wife, Nancy, "Don't breast-feed the baby; those breasts are *mine!*" Nancy called me for advice because she could not nurse her baby. "I get so nervous and Ariel is so squirmy, she won't suck; I just don't know what to do." Any wonder?

Many women have expressed concern over taking medication to ease pain after childbirth or to loosen their stools after a cesarean because they are concerned the medication will go into their breast milk. According to Susan, a La Leche League leader,

It is important to let the nursing staff know how very important
breast-feeding is to you and your baby. If you do need medication for pain, take it before the pain becomes excruciating. That
way you will be on top of the pain, and actually need less medication. The dosage should always be adjusted accordingly.
Then you should begin to nurse your baby as often as you can
or as often as your baby needs to eat or suck. (personal communication, August, 1994)

If you have complications or if your recovery is extremely difficult,
request that your partner or childbirth assistant hold your baby
close. The nurses in the nursery often have many babies to attend to
and cannot convey the message of love, security and closeness that
is your baby's birthright.

Bestfeeding: Getting Breastfeeding Right for You, by Mary Renfrew, Chloe Fisher and Suzanne Arms (1990), offers an innovative
approach to breast-feeding. The book has been designed to allow
you to find help quickly on positioning your baby. It gives suggestions for proper feeding and offers ten basic steps for breast-feeding
in English and Spanish. After a cesarean section, it is particularly important for you to position your body comfortably to ease nursing
and prevent pain. Positioning yourself on a flat bed may be more
comfortable. Have the side rails of the hospital bed up, and use them
to hold on to as you carefully roll onto your side. Request lots of pillows to cushion your body. Ask the nurse to place them wherever
you need extra support. Put two pillows under your head, and a couple of pillows between your knees. Then place your baby on her side
facing you and you are ready to start nursing. The two of you can
even fall asleep this way, cuddling in each other's closeness.

I slept this way with my first baby. I refused to allow anyone to
take her out of my room. I felt it was vital that she stay with me or
her father. Most of the time while I slept, so did she. Unfortunately,
the pain medication that I needed to take after my cesarean made her
a little bit groggy. I do remember at least one time when I was in
quite a bit of pain and I wanted desperately to sleep. My baby was
awake and fussy. My husband was not nearby at the moment, so I
called in the nurse. I told her that I believed babies need constant unconditional love and reassurance in their new and strange environment. I explained that my baby needed to be held and not left
isolated in the nursery, with no one around to comfort her. I asked
the nurse if she had time to help me out. She lovingly took my

daughter and held her for quite some time until a family friend arrived; she then placed the baby in my friend's arms, while I gratefully slept.

Cohen and Estner (1983) write,

> Let us not allow ourselves to schedule feedings or limit nursings the way our labors are scheduled and limited. Let's not permit artificial supplements into our babies' bodies the way artificial labor stimulants are pumped into our own. Let us allow our natural mothering hormones to flow as breastfeeding is established. Let's not leave our babies to cry; as many women are left during labor. Let's give our babies the very best we have to give. The very best does not come in bottles from an animal that has three stomachs, chews its cud, and says, "Moo." (p. 206)

Some women have expressed feelings that they are being manipulated by their newborn or that this new baby has taken over their lives. The concept of feeding on *demand* can foster those feelings. That is why I recommend that women feed their babies on *request*. Adults eat and drink at will, often grabbing a drink of water, a cup of coffee or an apple at odd times of the day or night. Why do people insist that new babies be on a schedule? Being fed, held, talked to, cooed at and allowed to suck are the primal needs of a newborn. Who are we to say they can only have food and attention every four to six hours?

Currently in our society there are numerous approaches and belief systems to parenting. Studies show that unconditional love and positive parenting make an enormous difference in the development and well-being of the whole child—not to mention the sanity of the parents! Whichever approach or belief system you may hold, the basic innate need to love and be loved unconditionally is universal. Why refrain from giving it to a newborn baby?

Chapter 15

Circumcision: A Question of Protecting Body Rights

Marilyn Fayre Milos

Marilyn Fayre Milos, a Registered Nurse and the Founder and Executive Director of the National Organization of Circumcision Information Resource Centers (NOCIRC), is an internationally recognized authority on the practices of male circumcision and female genital mutilation. Her work is based on the inalienable right of every human being to an intact body.

After organizing the First International Symposium on Circumcision in 1989, she produced a documentary videotape on the event and, as guest co-editor of The Truth Seeker Magazine, *documented the core proceedings of the symposium.*

Ms. Milos has appeared on many radio and television programs including Donahue *and* Nightline. *Her work has been covered by numerous newspapers and magazines. In addition to producing an educational videotape, "Informed Consent," she is also the editor of the* NOCIRC *Newsletter. Her published works include "Circumcision: What I Wish I Had Known," "Circumcision: A Medical or a Human Right's Issue?" (1992), "Circumcision Male" and "Circumcision Surgery" (1993), and "Circumcision: Male—Effects Upon Human Sexuality" (1994). Her own book on circumcision is forthcoming.*

In 1988, the California Nurses' Association presented Ms. Milos with the Maureen Ricke Award "for her dedication and unwavering commitment to righting a wrong" and "for her work on behalf of children to raise public consciousness about America's most unnecessary surgery." Ms. Milos says "circumcision, like other unnecessary surgeries such as cesareans, is clearly a violation of body integrity."

Every newborn infant is special. Amazing is the newborn in that he is born intact with eyes that see, ears that hear, a nose that smells, and skin that feels. The healthy newborn infant has needs to be loved, to be held, to be talked to, to be touched. He does not need to have the agonizing pain of part of his body surgically removed without any anesthesia inflicted upon him for non-existing health reasons. He does not need to be circumcised for reasons of religion or social customs or superstition. An ancient ignorance has made the care of the newborn's penis quite complicated when it should be quite simple. 'Leave it alone' is the commandment to all parents and health workers that should be heard around the world.

                                        Paul M. Fleiss, M.D.

Throughout history, people around the world have practiced circumcision. For some, such as Jews and Moslems, it has been a religious ritual; for others, as in Australia and Africa, it has been a puberty rite.

Circumcision is the surgical removal of the skin that normally covers and protects the head, or glans, of the penis. At birth, the penis is covered with a continuous layer of skin extending from the pubis to the tip of the penis, where the foreskin (prepuce) folds inward on itself, creating a double protective layer of skin over the glans penis. The inner lining of the prepuce is mucous membrane and serves to keep the surface of the glans penis (also mucous membrane) soft, moist and sensitive.

The surgery, usually performed on baby boys within the first few days of life, is often considered "routine." The most popular methods of circumcision, the Gomco clamp and the Plastibell procedure, differ somewhat in technique and instrumentation, but the effects on the penis and the baby are basically the same.

For the surgery, the baby is strapped spread-eagle to a plastic board with his arms and legs immobilized by Velcro straps. A nurse scrubs his genitals with an antiseptic solution and places a surgical drape—with a hole in it to expose his penis—across his body. The doctor grasps the tip of the foreskin with one hemostat (a scissor-like instrument used for grasping or compressing tissue) and inserts another hemostat between the foreskin and the glans. (In ninety six percent of newborns, these two structures are attached to one another by a continuous layer of epithelium, which protects the sensitive glans from urine and feces in infancy and childhood.) The foreskin, then, is torn from the glans. The hemostat is used to crush an area of the foreskin lengthwise, thus preventing bleeding when the doctor cuts through the tissue to enlarge the foreskin opening. This allows insertion of the circumcision instrument. The foreskin is crushed against this device and amputated.

While eighty five percent of the world's male population is not circumcised, circumcision is the most commonly performed surgical procedure in America, where sixty percent of newborn males undergo this operation annually. In the western states, however, sixty percent of boys are now left intact, indicating the trend away from this unnecessary surgery. Circumcision reached its peak of eighty five to ninety percent during the 1960s and 1970s. The United States is the only remaining country that routinely circumcises the majority of its male infants for non-religious and non-medical reasons.

Circumcision began in the English-speaking countries during the mid-1800s, supposedly to prevent masturbation, which was believed to cause many diseases. Since that time, various rationales have perpetuated its practice, but all of these—including the claims that circumcision prevents penile and cervical cancers and the spread of venereal disease—have been disproved (Wallerstein, 1980). The fear of increased urinary tract infections (UTIs) in intact boys comes from flawed studies that have been refuted. Before the unfortunate publication of these studies, female infants had the greater risk of UTI. Circumcision was never recommended as a prophylactic treatment for baby girls, although females, like their brothers, were also circumcised to prevent masturbation. As for hygiene, the American Academy of Pediatrics assured parents that "soap and water offer all the advantages of circumcision without the risk of surgery."

Although rarely mentioned, circumcision has the same risks as any other surgery: hemorrhage, infection, mutilation and death. Circumcised men have begun to speak up about the botched circumcisions that have left their penises with extensive scars, missing hunks or slices, skin bridges, curvatures, decreased sensitivity and, all too often, sexual dysfunction. These men describe the physical and psychological scars they carry as the result of an excruciatingly painful elective surgery to which they did not consent.

Until recently, it was generally assumed that babies did not feel pain during circumcision. This, in fact, may have been true when mothers were routinely anesthetized for birth and babies were routinely circumcised in the delivery room. As recipients of their mother's medication, babies may not have felt the pain of the surgery or were so drugged that they were unable to react to it.

But, with the advent of natural childbirth, things changed. Babies screamed during the surgery as the doctor literally crushed, sliced, clamped and amputated the foreskin—all without anesthesia. Why didn't anyone notice the screams when they could hear them, as they watched babies turn blue, vomit, or defecate during the surgery? Perhaps it was because the medical community had determined that responses to pain were reflexive, that perception of pain was not localized or present or that babies had a high pain threshold as an adaptive modality to what was considered the pain of birth. We should also consider Dr. Wilhelm Reich's observation that anyone who has repressed a feeling in himself will be incapable of recognizing the expression of that same feeling in someone else, making empathy impossible.

Some health professionals believed that babies were merely crying because they were tied down. However, in the research of Fran Porter, cries were measured on laboratory instruments so that the intensity of pain could be objectively analyzed. Porter's studies (1986) accurately identified cries associated with crushing, clamping and cutting of the foreskin as the most painful parts of the procedure. With this new information, excuses could no longer be used for the babies' dramatic response to the pain of circumcision.

Scientific research had to validate what anyone with common sense and empathy was able to recognize. In 1988, the American Medical Association declared the obvious: babies do feel pain. A special article, "Pain and Its Effects in the Human Neonate and Fetus," helped to bring the issue into focus. Drs. Anand and Hickey reported on the many studies that demonstrated the physiologic changes—cardiovascular, respiratory, hormonal and metabolic—as well as the behavioral changes—simple motor responses, facial expressions and crying—associated with pain. They reported on the complex behavioral responses seen after circumcision such as alterations in sleep-wake cycles that are indicative of prolonged stress and altered arousal levels.

Referring to Marshall's study, "Circumcision: Effects upon Newborn Behavior," which recognized changed behavioral states in infants for more than twenty-two hours after circumcision, Anand and Hickey wrote: "It was therefore proposed that such painful procedures may have prolonged effects on the neurologic and psychosocial development of neonates."

With regard to the memory of pain in neonates and how it affects them, Anand and Hickey report, "In the short term, these behavioral changes may disrupt the adaptation of newborn infants to their post-natal environment, the development of parent-infant bonding, and feeding schedules." The pain of circumcision clearly disrupts all of these. Furthermore, this violation of physical and emotional safety and the resultant interference with normal bonding disturb the most basic levels of trust.

"Baby's basic trust, emotional trust, in mother and the environment has been seriously compromised," said developmental neuropsychologist Dr. James Prescott in his presentation to the Third Annual Symposium on Circumcision (May, 1994, College Park, Maryland).

> Depression sets in and that is the beginning of sociopathy and psychopathy. We talk about empathy and compassion. How can you develop empathy and compassion when you're abandoned emotionally? That is what happens at a very deep primitive level.

In her talk at the Second International Symposium on Circumcision (May 3, 1991, San Francisco, California), psychiatrist Rima Laibow, M.D., reaffirmed Eric Erickson's model of the mother as responsible for the successful completion of her infant's first developmental task: establishing trust.

> An infant does retain significant memory traces of traumatic events. When a child is subjected to intolerable, overwhelming pain, it conceptualizes mother as both participatory and responsible regardless of mother's intent . . . the perception of the infant of her culpability and willingness to have him harmed is indelibly emplaced. The consequences for impaired bonding are significant.

Circumcision is insidious because it is experienced during the pre-verbal state, and the memory exists in feelings rather than words. However, some men claim never to have forgotten the experience. "It was like a giant bird landed on my stomach and disemboweled me with his talons. I can still feel the excruciating pain." Others, who have relived their circumcisions through hypnotherapy or psychotherapy, also describe the experience as terrifying and excruciatingly painful.

Unfortunately, not all men commit to such self-evaluation. It may be easier to live in denial than to face the atrocious act we commit on more than one million baby boys each year, an act that has affected the majority of men in the United States. In deciding not to circumcise his son, one father wrote:

> What was so difficult in leaving my son intact was not that my son would feel different in a locker room, but that I would feel different from him. I would then have to accept that I'm an amputee from the wars of a past generation.

Nevertheless, not all circumcised men were glad to be without their foreskin, even if they "matched" their circumcised peers. Many would have preferred to have all their body parts and tell us that, even as children, they could have understood a simple and honest explanation, perhaps one they will tell their own sons:

> Circumcision was thought to be important for health reasons when your dad and brothers were born, but now we know better. Your foreskin is normal and healthy. Circumcision is not necessary.

One man told his friends that, when his son asked why his penis was different, he would tell his boy that he had the "new, improved model!"

In spite of parental fears of a son's being different—never a concern when the practice was instituted and circumcised boys had intact fathers—some intact men reveal other feelings.

> I've been against circumcision since I first heard of the procedure when I was about nine. That was 33 years ago. By the time I was 14, I realized I was a member of a distinct minority—owners of a foreskin. I used to avoid having other boys see my foreskin for fear they'd be jealous of me. I felt sorry for my classmates and didn't want them to be reminded of what had been done to them.

It must not be easy for our circumcised fathers, brothers, husbands and sons to learn what the rest of the world has never questioned: the foreskin is normal, healthy, protective, sexually functioning tissue that provides the skin necessary for a full erection. Furthermore, a Canadian pathologist, Dr. John Taylor, describes the foreskin as being to the penis what the fingertip is to the finger. In other words, the nerve endings in the foreskin are exquisitely sensitive. Men are coming to terms with their loss, recognizing the violent violation of their bodies when they were too little to defend themselves and trying to heal their wounds. Men are seeking to become survivors rather than remain victims.

As the only woman presenter on a six-member panel at a Seattle seminar (November, 1992), I felt I was passing the torch. The five male panelists discussed circumcision from the male perspective. When it was my turn, I talked about my own experience—realizing the horror of the circumcisions my own babies had endured and the politics I've encountered as a woman ("Why are you sticking your nose in men's business?"), as a mother ("You just do this work because you feel guilty as the mother of three circumcised sons") and as a nurse ("You're upsetting the patients! You're fired!"). As a woman, a mother and a nurse, I closed my presentation with a quotation from Miriam Pollack's presentation in Seattle, Washington, two weeks earlier, entitled *Circumcision: Judaism, Feminism and Psychology.*

> We need to support and affirm men's struggle to revision the old notion of masculinity which is rooted in fear of women. . . . We invite men to explore ways to ritualize and celebrate masculinity and the critical passages of male bonding in ways that are life affirming, non-violent and protective of the sacred wholeness of men.

During the showing of a circumcision videotape that followed, men in the audience wept. Jed Diamond, a men's rights activist and psychotherapist, acknowledged the pain men were experiencing and then directed the audience toward healing. These men, I thought, would be survivors. The collective pain of generations could actually stop with them.

As women, circumcision is our concern too. Just as we protect the integrity of our own bodies during birth against intrusive measures such as use of IVs and fetal heart monitors, episiotomies or cesarean sections unless they are absolutely necessary, we must also protect the integrity of the bodies of our sons. Before males know they have a penis to protect, women know that they have a baby to protect. And, if our males were not protected from routine neonatal circumcision, then it is imperative that we protect them now. If they need to cry or to share their feelings, we need to provide a safe environment for them to do so. In that way, healing can take place and repressed anger will not be unconsciously projected onto the next generation.

When in Doubt . . .

Tell the truth.

Keep your promises.

Take responsibility
for your own experience.

Ask for what you need.

Pay attention.

Breathe.

Author unknown

Chapter 16

A Womb of Love
Andrea Frank Henkart

My innermost goal has been to affect healing of birth in a loving and gentle way. Our first experience in this life is through birth. Therefore, I feel that creating an understanding of the importance of a loving and gentle birth experience is vital for this healing. Over the years, I have assisted many women in having healthier, happier babies. These women had high quality births because they took responsibility; they learned how to trust themselves, their bodies and their babies. They learned how to communicate with their care providers and how to stand up for themselves.

Women today are faced with many challenges when deciding to have a baby. There is so much to learn, so much to prepare for and so many decisions to make. Unfortunately, women are not receiving all the information and support that should be made available to them. We deserve to know all of the options available so we can make conscious, educated choices in childbirth.

Childbirth has become shrouded in technocracy. The majority of women in America give birth in the hospital. The United States has one of the highest cesarean section rates in the world. Birth by major abdominal surgery is on the rise, and repeat cesareans are predominately elective and unnecessary. Despite the sophisticated, expensive equipment used in childbirth today, America still ranks very low in maternal and infant morbidity and mortality rates. Obstetricians continue to cut women open despite research that advocates the safety of vaginal birth and vaginal birth after cesarean. Cesareans are most often performed due to medical interventions, invasive procedures, obstetric interference, and fear of the natural birthing process.

Women are taught to believe that a drugged birth or a cesarean birth is easier and safer than a non-invasive vaginal birth. What is worse, many women are unaware of the risks and complications inherent in these procedures. Vaginal delivery may not always be the magical experience women hope it will be. However, complications from vaginal delivery occur less often and are far less severe than complications from cesarean surgery. Our own hormones for stimulating strong contractions have all but been replaced by synthetic drugs. Slicing the perineum instead of stretching it seems to be the trend in "getting the baby out" safely.

The medical society seems to believe that childbirth is impossible without the use of tubes, machines, drugs and knives. Women have been giving birth since the beginning of time. Can it be that suddenly our bodies do not work? Or is it our belief system that tells us someone else will rescue us and get our babies out for us? Doctors deliver the babies instead of women giving birth to them.

Our culture promotes in-hospital childbirth classes with an emphasis on the demystification of painkillers and techniques for breathing, as if teaching an already breathing person to inhale and exhale will eliminate the fear, anxiety and lack of confidence so many women bring into their birth experience. Men are often equally as vulnerable when the women they care about are in the throes of labor. Partners are encouraged to "coach" the laboring woman. In sports, a coach yells from the sidelines, determines the way the game will be played and makes snap judgments. On the contrary, couples need team encouragement, guidance and loving support during the birth process. A supportive, patient and loving birth assistant who believes in the normal, natural process of childbirth should be part of the team as an assistant to the emerging family.

Giving birth requires great energy. Nourishment assists the body's ability to function at its peak. Yet women in America are consistently deprived of food and drink during labor. Ordered to wear revealing hospital gowns and lie down in bed, subjected to numerous vaginal exams (often by a receiving line of well-meaning interns), hooked up to tubes and monitors "just in case," tied to the bed by fetal monitors, unable to move around freely, women are stripped of their dignity and often do not even realize it. It is this kind of treatment that promotes feelings of helplessness, dis-ease and negativity toward the natural process of childbirth.

Hospitals are institutions devoted to healing the sick. A woman in labor is not sick! Men, who do not know what giving birth feels like, are the majority of obstetricians. Can a man truly know what a woman feels in labor just by studying it in medical school? Women are given drugs to quiet them down and drugs to get their uterus going. They are told when to breathe and when to push the baby out. From the onset of pregnancy, we are warned about the possible interventions and inherent dangers of bringing a baby into the world. The pelvis is not a rigid confined space, nor is labor a rigid, learned skill to be managed by timetables and outside interference.

We are taught to be afraid of labor and to be afraid of the pain. Labor pains are not like the pain of a broken arm or menstrual cramps. It is pain with a purpose. Each wave that comes over your body brings your baby closer to being in your arms. If women would view each wave of contraction as one individual wave that has to be felt, welcomed, accepted and released, then labor would no longer be an experience to fear but would become a powerful, self-awakening experience.

What examples can we show our sons and daughters about the miracle of conception, pregnancy, labor, delivery and parenting if we are "sick" during pregnancy, request drugs during labor and feel numb during delivery? How can a woman consciously and respectfully parent if she is absolved from all feelings during childbirth? We must awaken from our numbed state of awareness for our own sake and for the future of our children. Technology does not have to destroy the emotional intensity of childbirth. As givers of life, women must maintain a sense of trust, honesty and self confidence.

As women, we are the birth givers and we are the change makers. We hold the power as new life passes through our limbs. There is a knowing deep inside that we can hear if we are quiet enough. Our inner voice will guide us as another soul is brought to life. Childbirth is a time for joy, for celebration, for respect and for love. As a baby emerges, so the family is born; a miracle to be treasured and honored for a lifetime.

Appendix A

Questions to Ask Your Care Provider

Be sure you ask appropriate questions to determine that your care provider's beliefs and philosophy about childbirth are compatible with your personal beliefs. Remember, if your care provider gets angry when you ask questions, you have the option to change doctors or midwives at any time. Do not limit your questions to those listed here, but use them as a guideline to formulate questions that work for you and the type of birth experience you want to have.

- What is your cesarean section rate?
- How do you see your role during my pregnancy, labor and birth?
- In what kind of setting do you currently practice: hospital, home or birth center?
- What procedures do you consider to be routine or mandatory?
- What procedures can be waived?
- How long do you wait before inducing labor?
- What drugs do you use to induce labor?
- How do you monitor labor of low-risk and high-risk women?
- What is your protocol regarding:
    - Routine prenatal testing
    - Ultrasound

–External cephalic version if the baby is breech (turning the fetus to a head-first position after thirty seven weeks)

-Trial of labor for VBACs

–Premature rupture of membranes

–Amniotomy

–Routine use of electronic fetal monitor (EFM)

–Routine use of internal fetal monitor (IFM)

–Pitocin augmentation

–Episiotomy

- How will you help me to avoid situations that may otherwise warrant the use of various interventions?
- What is your opinion on drugs used to induce labor?
- In what way do you promote VBAC?
- Do you follow policies designed to lower the local and national cesarean rates?
- How will you support me in avoiding an unnecessary cesarean section?
- Do you use fetal blood sampling or fetal stimulation tests to confirm fetal distress indicated by EFM?
- Will you treat me with respect throughout my labor and delivery? In what ways will you do that?
- How is the baby handled at birth and immediately after the birth?
- Will you treat my newborn with reverence and respect?
- What are your fees and will my insurance cover them?
- What is your personal philosophy about "natural childbirth?"

Ideas for Your Birth Plan

Create the plan that works best for you. Write in what is appropriate for your specific needs or use the sample suggested here. *Remember to leave room for the care provider's initials.* What they do not agree upon can always be drawn up as a waiver in the hospital. Find the inner strength to create the birth you want!

OUR BIRTH PLAN

We firmly believe in the normal, natural process of childbirth and fully expect our child's birth to be free of complications. As it may be difficult to make conscious decisions during labor and delivery, we are providing this list of requests to eliminate the possibility of any confusion or misunderstanding at the time of our baby's birth. We have provided space for initials if the request is within your parameters. Please inform us if a consent form or waiver is required.

Labor

Unrestricted mobility and freedom to move

Minimum of internal exams

Eating and drinking as desired

No routine use of fetal monitor

Friends, relatives, siblings present as requested by mother

Delivery

No routine catheterization

Positioning during pushing up to mother

No time limit for pushing

No routine episiotomy; try massage, warm compresses and support to perineum

Mother allowed to touch baby's head as it crowns

Baby to be placed on mother's abdomen immediately after birth

Partner to cut umbilical cord after it stops pulsing

After Birth

Baby care done on mother. Skin to skin contact

Baby to stay with parents

Vitamin K decision will be made

If recovery room is necessary, partner and baby go as a family

Delay non-essential routines and tests

Breast-feeding as baby desires

Postpartum

No routine separation of mother and baby

Siblings and family visits

All procedures/medications discussed with parents

24 hour rooming-in

Baby to sleep in bed with mother for warmth and breast-feeding ease

No bottles; breast-feeding as baby requests

If Cesarean Is Necessary

Surgery only after labor begins

Partner present, even if general anesthesia is necessary

Mother allowed to wear glasses or contact lenses

Mother's hands free to hold baby immediately after operation

Mother allowed to see placenta if so desired

Childbirth assistant present during surgery for support

Mother allowed to see baby and breast-feed in recovery room

If Baby Requires ICU

Partner to go along with baby

Parents involved in care of baby

Mother's milk only (will pump if necessary)

Mother allowed to hold baby

If Complications Arise

All previous requests to be honored to the fullest extent possible

Appendix C

Affirmations for Childbirth Preparation

Pick one or two affirmations, or create your own. Write each affirmation ten to twenty times every day, staying in the present tense. You may want to record any resistance that may arise as you watch your own progression. Continue working with your affirmations daily until they become completely integrated into your consciousness. Stay positive!

- It is safe for me to do things differently.
- It is safe for me to be in my body.
- I no longer have to withhold to survive.
- I forgive my mother for being afraid of childbirth.
- I no longer need drugs to feel alive.
- I forgive my obstetrician completely.
- I forgive myself completely.
- I forgive everyone and everything at my previous birth that was unpleasant.
- Having a baby is safe and easy for me right now!
- My intuitive wisdom knows just what to do.
- The more I relax and breathe, the more I open.
- My vagina and perineum can stretch to enormous proportions.
- I open to receive life.
- My baby knows the exact right time to be born.

- My body and my baby are safe, even though I may feel afraid.
- I give birth easily and effortlessly.
- I am a wonderful, gentle mother.
- My baby is healthy and perfect.

Appendix D

Things You Can Do to Avoid Unnecessary Cesareans

The International Cesarean Awareness Network has set up the following guidelines:

Before Labor

Read and educate yourself. Attend classes, groups and workshops inside and outside of the hospital environment.

Research and prepare a birth plan. Submit copies to your hospital or birth facility, doctor or midwife, and labor support persons.

Interview more than one care provider. Ask key questions, see what their responses are and how your probing influences their attitudes. Are they defensive or are they pleased by your interest?

Ask your care provider if there is a set time limit for labor and second stage pushing. See what he/she feels can interfere with the normal process of labor.

Tour more than one birth facility, note their differences, and ask about their cesarean rate, VBAC protocol, etc. Become aware of your rights as a pregnant woman.

Find a labor support person. Interview more than one, look for someone who has attended several births and has background

Reprinted by permission, 1993

experience with normal, non-interventive birth. Good labor support can significantly reduce the need for a cesarean.

Help ensure a healthy baby and mother by eating a well-balanced diet. Eating foods rich in protein, vitamins, and minerals can prevent complications in pregnancy, labor and delivery. Salt restriction is not recommended during pregnancy. Salt food to taste.

If your baby is breech, ask your care provider about "tilt-position" exercises, external version (turning of the baby) and vaginal breech delivery. You may want to seek a second opinion.

If you have had a prior cesarean, seriously consider and explore the option of vaginal birth after cesarean (VBAC). According to the October 1988 VBAC guidelines from the American College of Obstetricians and Gynecologists, VBAC is safer in most cases than a scheduled repeat cesarean. Up to 80% of women with prior cesarean sections can go on to deliver their subsequent babies vaginally.

During Labor

Stay at home as long as possible. Walk and change positions frequently. Labor in the position most comfortable to you. Remember, squatting can help. Do not labor or give birth flat on your back, as the weight of the baby on the vena cava (a major blood vessel in the mother's abdomen) can decrease the blood supply and oxygen to your body.

Continue to eat and drink lightly, especially during early labor. The uterus is a muscle, and like all muscles, it must be nourished to work effectively.

Avoid Pitocin augmentation for a slow labor. If your labor is progressing slowly, you may want to try nipple stimulation. Nipple stimulation and loving caresses may also get your labor going when you are past your due date. Remember, delivering past your due date and/or a slow labor may be normal for you.

If your bag of water breaks, don't let anyone do a vaginal examination (to avoid the risk of infection), unless medically indicated for a specific reason. Discuss with your care provider about how to monitor for signs of infection.

Recent studies have shown that the routine use of continual electronic fetal monitoring contributes to an increase in cesareans without related improvements in fetal outcome. Request the use of a fetoscope or perhaps just an initial monitoring strip upon admission to your birthing facility.

Epidurals and other anesthesia can slow down labor and can cause complications for the mother and baby. If you do have an epidural and are having trouble pushing effectively, let the epidural wear off and then resume pushing.

Do not arrive at the hospital too early. If you are still in the early stages of labor when you get to the birthing facility, instead of being admitted, walk around the hospital or go home and rest.

Find out the risks and benefits of routine and emergency procedures before you're faced with them. When faced with any procedure, find out why it is being used in your case, what are the short and long term effects on your baby, and what are your other options.

Remember, nothing is absolute. If you have doubts, trust your instincts. Do not be afraid to assert yourself. Accept responsibility for your requests and decisions.

Appendix E

Sources of Further Information

The American Academy of Husband Coached Childbirth (AAHCH)
(Bradley Method)
P.O. Box 5224
Sherman Oaks, CA 91413-5224
(800) 42-BIRTH or (800) 423-2397

The American College of Nurse Midwives (ACNM)
1522 K Street, N.W., Suite 1120
Washington, DC 20005
(202) 347-5445

Association for Childbirth at Home, International (ACHI)
116 S. Louise
Glendale, CA 91205
(213) 663-4996

Birth & Life Bookstore
P.O. Box 70625
Seattle, WA 98107-0625
(206) 789-4444

Birth Works
42 Tallwood Drive
Medford, NJ 08055
(609) 953-9380

California Association of Midwives (CAM)
P.O. Box 417854
Sacramento, CA 95841
(800) 829-5791

Cascade Birthing Catalog
P.O. Box 12203
Salem, OR 97309
(503) 378-7545

Cesarean Support, Education, and Concern (C/SEC, Inc.)
22 Forest Road
Framingham, MA 01701
(508) 877-8266

Consumer Advocates for the Legalization of Midwifery (CALM)
P.O. Box 922
Davis, CA 95617
(916) 756-5906

Hahnemann Medical Clinic (A Homeopathic Medical Clinic)
828 San Pablo Avenue
Albany, CA 94706
Clinic: (510) 524-3711/Pharmacy: (510) 527-3003

Homeopathic Educational Services
2124 Kittridge Street
Berkeley, CA 94704
(800) 359-9051

Informed Homebirth/Informed Birth and Parenting
P.O. Box 3675
Ann Arbor, MI 48106
(313) 622-6857

International Cesarean Awareness Network, Inc. (ICAN) (formerly CPM-Cesarean Prevention Movement, Inc.)
P.O. Box 276
Clarks Summit, PA 18411-0726
(717) 585-ICAN
Call or write for a chapter near you.

International Childbirth Education Association (ICEA)
P.O. Box 20048
Minneapolis, MN 55420-0048
(800) 624-4934

John Gray Seminars
4364 East Corral Road
Phoenix, AZ 85044
(800) 821-3033 or (602) 345-8430

La Leche League International
P.O. Box 1209
Franklin Park, IL 60131-8209
(800) LA-LECHE

Midwives Alliance of North America (MANA)
P.O. Box 175
Newton, KS 67114
(316) 283-4543

Moonflower Birthing Supply
P.O. Box 128
Louisville, CO 80027
(303) 665-2120

Mothering Magazine
P.O. Box 1690
Santa Fe, NM 87504
(800) 424-3308 or (505) 984-8116

National Association of Childbirth Assistants (NACA)
205 Copco Lane "N"
San Jose, CA 95123
(800) 868-NACA

**National Association of Parents & Professionals for Safe
Alternatives in Childbirth (NAPSAC)**
P.O. Box 646
Marble Hill, MO 63764
(314) 238-2010

National Center for Homeopathy
1500 Massachusetts Ave. N.W., #42
Washington, DC 20005
(202) 223-6182

**National Organization of Circumcision Information Resource
Centers (NOCIRC)**
P.O. Box 2512
San Anselmo, CA 94979
(415) 488-9883

National Vaccination Information Center Dissatisfied Parents Together (DPT)
512 West Maple Avenue, #206
Vienna, VA 22180
(800) 909-SHOT

Natural Resources (a pregnancy, childbirth and early parenting resource center, catalog available)
4081 24th Street
San Francisco, CA 94114
(415) 550-2611

Bibliography and Suggested Reading List

ACOG President Warns against "Naked Self Interest." (1991). *Obstetrics & Gynecology News*. 26(12): 2, 35.

Althabe, O. (1969). Influence of the Rupture of Membranes on Compression of the Fetal Head During Labor. Paper Presented at Pan American Health Organization's Conference on Perinatal Factors Affecting Human Development. Washington, D.C.

American Academy of Pediatrics Ad Hoc Task Force on Circumcision. (1975). Report of the Ad Hoc Task Force on Circumcision. *Pediatrics*. 56(4): 610–611.

American College of Obstetrics and Gynecologists Committee on Obstetrics: Maternal and Fetal Medicine. *Guidelines for Vaginal Delivery after a Previous Cesarean Birth*. (October, 1988). Second Revision. Washington, D.C.: ACOG.

Anand, K.J.S., & Hickey, P. R. (1987). Pain and Its Effects in the Human Neonate and Fetus. *New England Journal of Medicine*. 317 (21): 1321–29.

Baker, J. P. (1980). *Hygeia: A Woman's Herbal*. Monroe, UT: Freestone.

Baker, J. P. (1986). *Prenatal Yoga & Natural Birth*. Berkeley, CA:. North Atlantic Books.

Baker, J. P., & Baker, F. (1986). *Conscious Conception: Elemental Journey Through the Labyrinth of Sexuality*. Monroe, UT: Freestone Publishing Company.

Balaskas, J. (1990). *Natural Pregnancy*. NY: Interlink Books.

Baldwin, R. (1986). *Special Delivery*. Berkeley, CA: Celestial Arts.

Bradley, R. (1965). *Husband-Coached Childbirth*. New York: Harper & Row.

Briggs, A. (1985). *Circumcision: What Every Parent Should Know*. North Garden, VA: Birth & Parenting Publications.

Brotanek, V., & Hodr, J. (1968). Fetal Distress after Artificial Rupture of Membrane. *American Journal of Obstetrics and Gynecology.* 101: 542.

Bullock, G. (1987). Apologies of a Reformed Obstetrician (unpublished).

Castro, M. (1992). *Homeopathy for Pregnancy, Birth and the First Year.* New York: St. Martin's Press.

Circumcision Why? (1985). Corte Madera, CA: National Organization of Circumcision Information Resource Centers.

Clemenson, N. (1993). Promoting Vaginal Birth after Cesarean Section. *American Family Physician.* 47 (1): 139–44.

Cohen, N. W. (1991). *Open Season: A Survival Guide for Natural Childbirth & VBAC in the 90s.* Westport, CT: Bergin & Garvey.

Cohen, N. W., & Estner, L. (1983). *Silent Knife: Cesarean Prevention & Vaginal Birth After Cesarean.* South Hadley, MA: Bergin & Garvey.

Consumer Advocates for the Legalization of Midwives (CALM). (1991). pamphlet. Davis, CA: CALM.

Coulter, H. L., & Fisher, B. L. (1985). *DPT: A Shot in the Dark.* Orlando, FL: Jovanovich.

Countryman, B. A. (1978). *Breastfeeding and Jaundice.* Franklin Park, IL: La Leche League.

Cragin, E. B. (1916). Conservatism in Obstetrics. *New York State Medical Journal.* 104: 1–3.

Creating the Birth You Want. (1992). *International Cesarean Awareness Network Pamphlet.* Syracuse, NY: ICAN.

Crolius, A. (Winter, 1992). Unexpected Encounters with Dutch Midwives. *Mothering Magazine.* 62: 83.

Cummings, S., & Ullman, D. (1984). *Everybody's Guide to Homeopathic Medicines.* Los Angeles, CA: Jeremy P. Tarcher.

Davis, E. (1988). *Energetic Pregnancy.* Berkeley, CA: Celestial Arts.

Davis, E. (1987). *Heart & Hands: A Midwife's Guide to Pregnancy & Birth.* Berkeley, CA: Celestial Arts.

Davis-Floyd, R. (1992). *Birth as an American Rite of Passage.* Berkeley, CA: University of California Press.

Davis-Floyd, R. (1993). "The Rituals of Hospital Birth." In *Conformity and Conflict: Readings in Cultural Anthropology.* 8th edition. David McCurdy, ed. New York: HarperCollins.

Davis-Floyd, R., & Sargent, C., eds. (in press). *Childbirth and Authoritative Knowledge: Cross-Cultural Perspectives.* Berkeley, CA: University of California Press.

Diamond, H., & Diamond, M. (1985). *Fit for Life.* New York: Warner Books.

Elliot, R. (1986). *Vegetarian Mother and Baby Book: A Complete Guide to Nutrition, Health and Diet During Pregnancy and After.* New York: Pantheon Books.

Evard, J. R., & Gold, E. M. (Nov. 1977). Cesarean Section and Maternal Mortality in Rhode Island: Incidence and Risk Factors 1965–1975. *Journal of Obstetrics & Gynecology.* 50: 594.

Fabin-Newmiller, K. (1991). *CALM Newsletter on Homebirth.* Davis, CA: Consumer Advocates for the Legalization of Midwives.

Flamm, B. (1990). *Birth after Cesarean, the Medical Facts.* New York: Prentice Hall Press.

Gabay, M., & Wolfe, S. (1994). *Unnecessary Cesarean Sections: Curing a National Epidemic.* Washington, D.C.: Public Citizen's Health Research Group.

Gaskin, I. M. (1990). *Spiritual Midwifery.* Summertown, TN: The Book Publishing Company.

Gaudenzi, G. (February 28, 1993). Che Affare il Cesareo. *L'Espresso.* Italy.

Gibbs, C. E. (1980). Planned Vaginal Delivery following Cesarean Section. *Clinical Obstetrics & Gynecology.* 23: 507–515.

Goer, H. (1995). *Obstetric Myths Versus Research Realities: A Guide to the Medical Literature.* Westport, CT: Bergin & Garvey.

Gray, J. (1992). *Men Are from Mars, Women Are from Venus.* New York: HarperCollins.

Gray, J. (1990). *Men, Women and Relationships: Making Peace with the Opposite Sex.* Hillsboro, OR: Beyond Words, Publishing, Inc.

Harris, R. P. (1879). A Study and Analysis of One Hundred Cesarean Operations Performed in the United States, During the Present Century, and Prior to the Year 1878. *American Journal of Medical Science.* 77: 43–65.

Harrison, M. (1982). *A Woman in Residence.* New York: Random House.

Hausknecht, R., & Heilman, J. R. (1991). *Having a Cesarean Baby.* New York: Plume Books.

Haverkamp, A. (1976). The Evaluation of Continuous Heart Rate Monitoring in High Risk Pregnancy. *American Journal of Obstetrics & Gynecology.* 125: 310.

Health Insurance Association of America. (1992). *Source Book of Health Insurance Data.* p. 74, Table 4.15.

How to Avoid an Unnecessary Cesarean. (1992). International Cesarean Awareness Network Pamphlet. Syracuse, NY: ICAN.

Jordan, B. (1993). *Birth in Four Cultures.* 4th Ed. Prospect Heights, IL: Waveland Press.

Kealoha, A. (1989). *Songs of the Earth.* Sebastopol, CA: Celestial Arts.

Kennell, J., Klaus, M., McGrath, S., Robertson, S., & Hinkley, C. (1991). Continuous Emotional Support During Labor in a U. S. Hospital: A Randomized Controlled Trial. *Journal of the American Medical Association.* 265: 2197–2201.

Kitzinger, S. (1993). *The Complete Book of Pregnancy and Childbirth.* New York: Alfred A. Knopf.

Kitzinger, S. (Nov. 1981). *Second Stage*. Lecture Given at Boston College. Boston, MA.

Kitzinger, S. (1987). *Some Women's Experiences of Epidurals*. London: National Childbirth Trust.

Klaus, M., Kennell, M. D., & Klaus, P. (1993). *Mothering the Mother*. New York: Addison-Wesley.

Klaus, M., & Klaus, P. (1994). *The Amazing Newborn*. Reading, MA: Addison-Wesley.

Klein, L. (1984). Cesarean Birth and Trial of Labor. *Female Patient* 9: 106–117.

Koehler, N. (1985). *Artemis Speaks: V.B.A.C. Stories & Natural Childbirth Information*. Occidental, CA: Jerald Brown.

Leboyer, F. (1975). *Birth without Violence*. New York: Alfred A. Knopf.

Lim, R. (1991). *After the Baby's Birth . . . A Woman's Way to Wellness*. Berkeley, CA: Celestial Arts.

Lowe, C. (1992). *Becoming a Childbirth Assistant: The Lowe Method*. San Jose, CA: Birth Support Providers.

Lowe, C. (1992). Technique. *The Childbirth Assistant Journal*. Vol. III, Issue III.

McKay, S., ed. (Spring, 1979). Physiologic Jaundice of the Newborn. Minneapolis, MI: *International Childbirth Education Association*. p. 3.

Malloy, M. H., et al. (Sept. 1989). C/Section: Does It Help Very Tiny Infants? *Journal of American Medical Association*. 262: 1475.

Malloy, M. H., Onstad, L., Wright E. National Institute of Child Health and Human Development Neonatal Research Network. (1991). The Effect of Cesarean Delivery on Birth Outcome in Very Low Birth Weight Infants. *Obstetrics and Gynecology*. 77 (4): 498–503.

Marshall, R. E. (1980). Circumcision: Effects upon Newborn Behavior. *Infant Behavioral Development*. 3: 1–14.

Mendelsohn, R. (1984). *How to Raise a Healthy Child . . . In Spite of Your Doctor*. Chicago: Contemporary Books.

Mendelsohn, R. (1981). *Mal(e) Practice*. Chicago: Contemporary Books.

Morales, K., & Inlander, C. (1991). *Take This Book to the Obstetrician with You*. Reading, MA: Addison-Wesley.

Moskowitz, R. (1992). *Homeopathic Medicines for Pregnancy and Childbirth*. Berkeley, CA: North Atlantic Books.

Murphy, H. (1976). Delivery following Caesarean Section. Ten Year's Experience at the Rotunda Hospital, Dublin. *Journal of the Irish Medical Association*. 69: 533–534.

Neustaedter, R. (1990). *The Immunization Decision: A Guide for Parents*. Berkeley, CA: North Atlantic Books.

Odent, M. (1984). *Birth Reborn*. New York: Pantheon Books.

Olkin, S. (1987). *Positive Pregnancy Fitness.* Garden City Park, NY: Avery.

Pain and Its Effects in the Human Neonate and Fetus. (1987). *New England Journal of Medicine.* 317: 1321–29.

Panos, M. B., & Heimlich, J. (1980). *Homeopathic Medicine at Home.* Los Angeles, CA: J. P. Tarcher.

Perez, P., & Snedeker, C. (1990). *Special Women: The Role of the Professional Labor Assistant.* Seattle: Pennypress.

Peterson, G. (1984). *Birthing Normally.* Berkeley, CA: Mindbody Press.

Petitti, D. B., Cefalo, R. C., Shapiro, S., & Whalley, P. (1982). In-Hospital Mortality in the United States: Time Trends and Relation to Method of Delivery. *Obstetrics and Gynecology.* 59: 6–11.

Porter, F. L., Miller, R. H., & Marshall, R. E. (1986). Neonatal Pain Cries: Effect of Circumcision on Acoustic Features and Perceived Urgency. *Child Development.* 57: 790–802.

The Pregnant Patient's Bill of Rights. (1986). Minneapolis, MN: International Childbirth Education Association.

Quilligan, E. J. (1983). Controlling the High C-Section Rate. *Contemporary Obstetrics and Gynecology.* January: 221.

Rates of Cesarean Delivery-United States, 1991. (1993). *Morbidity and Mortality Weekly Report.* 42 (15): 285–89.

Renfrew, M., Fisher, C., & Arms, S. (1990). *Bestfeeding: Getting Breastfeeding Right for You.* Berkeley, CA: Celestial Arts.

Richards, L. B. (1987). *The Vaginal Birth after Cesarean Experience.* South Hadley, MA: Bergin & Garvey.

Robbins, J. (1987). *Diet for a New America.* Walpole, NH: Stillpoint.

Sandmire, H. F. (1993). Discussion in the *American Journal of Obstetrics and Gynecology.* 168: 1755–56.

Sears, W., & Sears, M. (1994). *The Birth Book: Everything You Need to Know to Have a Safe and Satisfying Birth.* NY: Little, Brown and Company.

Seidman, M. (1986). *A Guide to Polarity Therapy: The Gentle Art of Hands-on Healing.* North Hollywood, CA: Newcastle.

Shiloh, J. (1990). *Homeopathy for Birthing.* Sedona, AZ: Rocky Mountain Press.

Simkin, P., & Reinke, C. (1980). *Planning Your Baby's Birth.* Seattle: Pennypress.

Smith, T. (1984). *A Woman's Guide to Homeopathic Medicine.* Rochester, VT: Thorsons Publishing Group.

Speert, H. (1980). *Obstetrics and Gynecology in America: A History.* Baltimore: Waverly Press.

Stein, D. (1991). *The Goddess Celebrates.* Freedom, CA: Crossing Press.

Stoppard, M. (1993). *Conception, Pregnancy & Birth.* London: Dorling Kindersley.

Thevinin, T. (1987). *The Family Bed: An Age Old Concept in Childrearing.* Minneapolis: Avery Press.

U. S. Department of Health and Human Services. (1981). *Cesarean Childbirth.* Bethesda, MD: National Institutes of Health Publication No. 82-2076.

U. S. Department of Health and Human Services, Public Health Service, Centers for Disease Control, National Center for Health Statistics. (March, 1991). *Health United States 1990.* DHHS Pub. No. (PHS) 91-1232. Table 21.

U. S. Department of Health and Human Services, Public Health Service, Centers for Disease Control, National Center for Health Statistics, Vital and Health Statistics. (1990). Summary: National Hospital Discharge Survey. *Advance Data.* No. 210, Table 7, p. 7.

VanTuinen, I., & Wolfe, S. (1992). *Unnecessary Cesarean Sections: Halting a National Epidemic.* Washington, D.C.: Public Citizen's Health Research Group.

Wallerstein, E. (1980). *Circumcision: An American Health Fallacy.* New York: Springer Publishing Co.

Wallerstein, E. (1980). *The Circumcision Decision.* Seattle: Pennypress.

Wallerstein, Edward. (1986). *Circumcision: Information, Misinformation & Disinformation.* Corte Madera, CA:. National Organization of Circumcision Resource Centers.

Zorn, E. B. (1990). The Duping of America's Childbearing Women. *The Clarion.* 7(4): 1.

Index

acceptance, 59, 63, 65
ACOG, 21, 105, 132
acupressure, 22
acupuncture, 22
affirmations, 40, 87, 99
American Academy of Pediatrics, 143
American Medical Association, 144
amniocentesis, 46
anesthesia: epidural, 8, 14, 35, 81, 82, 83, 87, 104–5; general, 3, 24, 81, 82, 84
anesthesiologist, 20
assertiveness, 45

Bali, 127
bikini cut, 20
bilirubin, 135, 136
birth experiences, influences on, 117
birth plan, 39, 45, 46, 47, 56, 99, 137
birth script, 100
birth stories: America, 124; England, 123; Italy, 119; Japan, 120; Korea, 123; Philippines, 121, 125

birth team, 43
birthing room, 13
birthing stool, 104
bodies: as machines; 28; as things, 75
body memory, 74, 78, 79
body positioning in labor, 40, 67, 103, 104
body talk, 76, 78
body wisdom, 74, 75, 79, 80
Bradley, 63
breast-feeding, 11, 45, 67, 83, 129, 136, 137, 138, 139; to prevent jaundice, 4
breastmilk, medication in, 137
breathing techniques, 61, 63, 65, 150
breech birth, 21, 22, 41, 46
British statistics on homebirth, 41

C/SEC (Cesarean Support, Education, and Concern), 105
cancer: cervical, 143; penile, 143
care provider, 39, 41, 42, 46, 48, 107
cascade of intervention, 30, 31
cephalopelvic disproportion (CPD), 23

ceremony, 93–96
cervical dilation, 9, 13, 17, 32, 50, 105
Cesarean Prevention Movement (CPM), 6, 11
cesarean section, 17, 24, 81; complications from, 152; medical indications for, 21, 24, 89, 105; prevention, 42, 102; repeat statistics, 19, 20, 29; rooming-in recovery from, 45; unnecessary, 41, 89, 107
cesarean section cost: Bali, 128; United States, 21
cesarean section rate: Bali, 128; Holland, 118; Italy, 119; United States, 16, 19, 26, 34, 55, 151
childbirth, 26, 60, 62, 153; assistant, 42, 44, 45, 47, 48, 50, 51, 99, 100, 101, 137, 138, 152; classes, 43, 47, 62–64, 81, 99, 115, 118, 152; education, 45, 59–65, 118
chiropractic care, 22, 39
choices in childbirth, 46
circumcision, 46, 132; effects upon behavior, 144, 145; effects upon physiology, 144, 145; statistics, 143; surgery, 142, 143
communication skills, 41, 43, 45, 47, 50, 64, 100, 101, 107
conception, 153
conscious conception, 91
consumer advocacy, 63
continuous labor support, 42
cord prolapse, 23
core beliefs and values, 26, 27, 34–37
counseling, 100
cravings, 101
cultural beliefs, 118
cultural differences, 117
cultural process, 36, 60
cultural unlearning, 64

denial, 145
depression, 145–147
diaphragmatic breathing, 68
doula, 44
dreams, 88, 106
drug-induced hallucination, 10
due dates, 53
Dutch midwives, 22, 40, 52, 119
dystocia, 21, 23

electronic fetal monitor, 8, 14, 26, 29, 30, 31, 34, 51, 53–56, 102, 118, 152
emotional needs, 110
emotional support, 44, 58, 82, 88, 101, 110
emotional wounding, 33, 85
emotions, 110, 114
empathy, 144
empowerment in labor, 54
epidural: epidemic, 35; rate, 34;
episiotomy, 14, 26, 33, 40, 51–53, 56; rates, 41, 52, 87
erythromycin, 46, 131
exercise, 22, 47, 83, 84, 99
exhaustion, in labor, 14, 57, 64
external version, 22

family support, 100
fears, 2, 106, 117
feelings, 63, 106
fetal distress, 21, 23, 46, 50, 55
fetal heart rate, 23, 30, 43, 51, 55
fetoscope, 55, 56
forceps delivery, 32, 41, 42, 56, 119, 132
foreskin: function, 142, 146; protection, 142, 146; structure, 142, 146
four t's, the, 111
freebirth, 95–97

gas, after a cesarean, 11, 83, 84
gentle birth, 134, 151

glans penis, 142
Gomco clamp, 142

herbs, 22, 40
high risk pregnancy, 20, 55
holistic healing, 36
holistic mythology, 36
Holland, 22, 40, 52, 104, 118
homebirth, 6, 36, 37, 40, 41, 42,
    118; rate in Bali, Indonesia, 129;
    rate in Holland, 104, 118
homeopathy, 3, 22, 40, 54
hospital, 16, 28, 29, 32, 35; proce-
    dure, 51, 99; protocol, 17, 28,
    29, 32, 42, 50, 82, 151, 153
husband's role, 109
hypnosis, 40, 87, 99

iatrogenic prematurity, 17
ICAN (The International Cesarean
    Awareness Movement), 6, 14, 24,
    51, 88, 89, 105
infant mortality rate, 16, 18, 129
informed choice, 89, 151
institutions, 27–29
IV, 26, 27, 32, 33, 57, 104

jaundice, neonatal, 4, 11, 132, 135,
    136

Kegel, 52

labor, 7, 43, 49, 61, 64, 65; coach,
    42, 43, 44, 63, 152; pains, 75,
    153; support, 43, 44; time sched-
    ule for, 42, 50
Lamaze, 61–63
language of the body, 76, 78
lithotomy position, 32, 103

major abdominal surgery, 5, 15,
    16
malpractice suits, 34
management of the newborn, 46

massage, 22, 58, 68, 84
maternal distress, 50
maternal hypotension, 105
maternal-infant bonding, 42, 45,
    81, 82, 85, 145
maternal morbidity and mortality
    rate, 16, 151; in Bali, 129; in
    Holland, 118
meconium, 136
medical costs, 42
medical interventions, 42, 47, 50,
    62, 64
medical records, 100
medicated birth, 99, 106, 152
medication, 143
meditation, 68, 99
midwives, 7, 18, 28, 37, 39, 40–42,
    96, 123–124; in Bali, 128, 129;
    in Holland, 104, 118
morning sickness, 49
motherhood, 2, 49, 61
myth, 26

natural childbirth, 1, 33, 34, 88,
    99, 102, 152
newborn, 42, 131, 134, 139
non-invasive birth, 14
nourishment in labor, 152
nutrition, 40, 47

obstetrician, 39, 44, 45, 47, 151,
    153
Oxytocin, 54, 105

pain, 3, 60, 62–64, 143–145, 147;
    after a cesarean, 82–84; medica-
    tion, 26, 43, 136, 138, 152
parenting, 131, 139, 153
patience, 64
patriarchy, 32
pelvic tilt, 22
perfect baby syndrome, 17, 29
perineal massage, 33, 52
perineum, 40, 46, 51, 52, 152

Pitocin, 3, 14, 26, 29–31, 42, 50, 51, 53, 54, 136
placenta, 67, 105
placental problems, 21, 23
Plastibell, 142
polarity therapy, 10
postdate pregnancy, 46
postpartum care, 129
postpartum depression, 33
postpartum hemorrhage, 128
postural tilt, 22
pregnancy, 45, 74, 76, 153; and your relationship, 114
pregnant patient, 46
prenatal care, 3, 39, 40, 41, 44, 128
prenatal nutrition, 101
prenatal yoga, 58, 84, 91
prepuce. *See* foreskin
psychological healing, 85
psychotherapy, 87
purebirth, 1

rebirthing, 99
recovery, 81, 84, 87
relaxation, 58, 67, 68; techniques, 62–65
responsibility, 39, 89, 100
rites of passage, 26
ritual, 26, 27, 29, 30, 33, 36, 37, 91–93, 96, 97
rituals of hospital birth, 26, 27
rooming-in, 45
routine tests, 46, 134

scars, 94, 127, 128, 143
second stage pushing, 32, 40, 42, 46, 51, 103
self-esteem, 110
self-responsibility, 36
single mothers, 42
social support, 42
sonogram. *See* ultrasound
special needs, 42

standardization of American birth, 26
stillbirth, 41
stress, 67
Super Woman, 67
support groups, 87
surgical-vaginal birth, 14
surrender, 49
symbolic anthropology, 26
symbols, 27

talk, 112, 115
technical aspects of birth, 42
technocracy, 27, 33, 34, 151
technocratic myth, 28, 29, 31, 36, 37
technology, 6, 33, 78
time, 113, 115
touch, 111, 115
transverse lie, 21, 22
trauma, 91–93, 96, 132
trial of labor, 20, 39
trust, 65, 86, 112, 115, 118, 145, 151

ultrasound, 19, 31, 45, 53
unconditional love, 139
urinary tract infection, 143
uterine contractions, 61
uterine rupture, 20
uterus, 20, 62

vacuum extraction, 119, 132
vaginal birth, 152
VBAC (vaginal birth after cesarean), 6, 11, 19, 20, 45, 52, 56, 89, 99, 100, 102, 106
vertical incision, 20
visualization techniques, 22, 58, 67, 71, 72, 88, 89
vitamin K, 46, 132, 136

x-rays, 3

ABOUT THE EDITOR

ANDREA FRANK HENKART has an M.A. in Psychology from Sonoma State University. She is a holistic health educator, a certified childbirth educator, a certified professional childbirth assistant, and the cofounder and past president of the Marin County chapter of the International Cesarean Awareness Network. As an international public speaker and seminar leader, Ms. Henkart has over 18 years of teaching experience in the fields of health, childbirth, parenting, and personal growth. She is the author of *The Cesarean Challenge*.